the**facts**

Autism and Asperger Syndrome

SIMON BARON-COHEN

Professor of Developmental
Psychopathology,
Director,
Autism Research Centre,
Cambridge University,
Cambridge, UK.

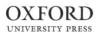

OXFORD
UNIVERSITY PRESS

OXFORD

UNIVERSITY PRESS

Great Clarendon Street, Oxford OX2 6DP

Oxford University Press is a department of the University of Oxford.
It furthers the University's objective of excellence in research, scholarship,
and education by publishing worldwide in

Oxford New York

Auckland Cape Town Dar es Salaam Hong Kong Karachi
Kuala Lumpur Madrid Melbourne Mexico City Nairobi
New Delhi Shanghai Taipei Toronto

With offices in

Argentina Austria Brazil Chile Czech Republic France Greece
Guatemala Hungary Italy Japan Poland Portugal Singapore
South Korea Switzerland Thailand Turkey Ukraine Vietnam

Oxford is a registered trade mark of Oxford University Press
in the UK and in certain other countries

Published in the United States
by Oxford University Press Inc., New York

British Library Cataloguing in Publication Data
Data available

Library of Congress Cataloguing in Publication Data
Data available

ISBN 978-0-19-850490-0 (Pbk.)

15

Typeset in Plantin
by Cepha Imaging Pvt. Ltd., Bangalore, India
Printed in Great Britain
on acid-free paper by
Ashford Colour Press, Gosport, Hampshire.

Contents

Acknowledgements

Autism is now an everyday word. It was not always so. When I started in this field 25 years ago, I would use a phrase such as 'autistic children' that some people would hear as 'artistic children', so unfamiliar were they with this word. That it is now a household word is in part due to the success of films such as *Rain Man*, which popularized at least one side of autism. This was the man who walked in an awkward fashion, who stammered and made little eye contact, but who noticed tiny details such as the number of match-sticks on the floor when a whole box of matches had spilt and who could remember which airlines had crashed, and the dates the crashes had happened, right through aviation history. His mind was like a look-up table of facts and figures. Such savant abilities are certainly seen in one subgroup of people with autism.

Autism has also become better known because of the remarkable success of parent-led lobbying groups in the UK and USA, and across the world, running an impressive campaign to ensure that politicians keep autism on the agenda for medical research funding, schools, clinical services and other forms of intervention.

In 1993, Patrick Bolton and I published a book in this series called *Autism: the facts*. In those days, classic autism (and such individuals may or may not have the savant or gifted abilities) was well diagnosed. In contrast, the other major subgroup (Asperger syndrome) was unheard of. These children and adults existed, but they were not recognized. These are the people who also have a form of autism, in that they have difficulties socializing and communicating, they also have narrowed interests and narrow attention to detail, and they also find unexpected change very difficult to manage. However, people with Asperger syndrome have normal IQ and no language delay.

Asperger wrote in German which may be why it went un-noticed for several decades, at least in the UK and the USA.

Although Lorna Wing wrote (in English) about Asperger syndrome in a journal article in 1981, her article took a while to be picked up by the clinical and research communities, let alone the policy makers and social services. Awareness of Asperger syndrome was helped when, in 1991, Uta Frith published an edited book called *Asperger Syndrome* (Cambridge University Press). However, it wasn't until 1994 that the American Psychiatric Association and the World Health Organization agreed that Asperger syndrome should be included in the major diagnostic classification systems of medical conditions.

For these reasons, *Autism: the facts* made no mention of Asperger syndrome, and the title of that book reflected that historical context. Our book became outdated for a number of other reasons. Aside from the lack of any mention of Asperger syndrome, the other two major features of that book that jar in the twenty-first century are the now incorrect notion that autism is quite rare (today we recognize it to be very common), and the terminology we used (terms such as 'mental handicap' and 'retardation' when today we would use terms such as 'learning difficulties'). In addition, *Austism: the facts* was no longer up-to-date in terms of the range of interventions on offer.

As a result, and given the fact that biomedical research into autism has now taken off, revealing a wealth of new data, in 2007 Oxford University Press invited me write a second edition called *Autism and Asperger syndrome: the facts*. I realized this would be an opportunity to revise the old book and to present a unified psychological theory of the autistic spectrum. This new book provides me with an opportunity to fill some gaps created by my previous books. Thus *Mindblindness* (MIT Press, 1995) only considered one aspect of autism and Asperger syndrome (the difficulties in attributing mental states to others). *The Essential Difference* (Penguin/Basic Books, 2003) only considered autism and Asperger syndrome in terms of its relationship to sex differences in the general population. *Prenatal Testosterone in Mind* (MIT Press, 2005) only considered one possible causal factor in autism (foetal androgens).

All of these books provide the reader with fragments of the puzzle. In this new book, I try to step back and paint the big picture of the psychology of autism. All the elements of autism spectrum conditions come together in an integrated psychological model. It is called the empathizing–systemizing model. Beyond the psychology of autism spectrum conditions, this book summarizes what we have learnt about the brain, genetics and interventions, so that someone who is looking for an introduction to autism and Asperger Syndrome can find it all in one place.

I am grateful to my colleagues and collaborators at the Autism Research Centre (ARC) in Cambridge who have helped me think through these ideas over the years, and to the families who have helped our research by taking part in our sometimes bizarre experiments. I hope this book gives something back to them. My collaborators Mike Lombardo, Sally Wheelwright, Greg Pasco, and Matthew Belmonte read the manuscript carefully to help me avoid the worst mistakes. Virginia Bovell and Adam Feinstein each have a child with autism, and they did me the enormous service of reading the draft of this book, when life with a child on the spectrum does not afford such time out. I owe them both a huge thank you. Michael Ellerman, Bernard Fleming, Matthew Downie, Richard Mills, Professor Sir Michael Rutter, and Dr Lorna Wing, provided valuable comments, for which I am indebted. Appendix 2 was kindly compiled by the National Autistic Society. Roger Freeman kindly pointed out typos in the first edition which have been corrected here.

I am also grateful to Bridget Lindley, who has worked for several decades to get rights for families whose child has become entangled in the child protection process, who has taught me the value of clear and accessible information as a way of empowering families under stress. I owe a debt to my three children, Sam, Kate and Robin. Long after they had gone to bed they could hear me tapping away at my computer. I am glad that academic life allowed me the flexibility to be a hands-on parent by day and a scholar by night. It meant we had plenty of fun, playful times, and they remained very good-natured in tolerating my own narrow focus of attention at night. Finally, I am full of respect for the many people with autism and Asperger syndrome I have met, and their families, who have shared their experience with me and who patiently taught me what little I know.

Figure acknowledgements

Figure 2.2, p17. Photo of Leo Kanner, MD is reproduced courtesy of Johns Hopkins Medical Institutions.

Figure 2.3, p19. Photo of Bruno Bettelheim is reproduced courtesy of the Special Collections Research Center, University of Chicago Library.

Figure 2.4, p20. Photo of Professor Niko Tinbergen is reproduced courtesy of the Tinbergen family.

Figure 2.7, p23. Photo of Professor Hans Asperger is reproduced courtesy of Dr Maria Asperger Felder.

Figure 3.2 and **Figure 3.3** are reproduced from Baron-Cohen et al, 'The Autism-Spectrum Quotient (AQ): Evidence from Asperger Syndrome/High-Functioning Autism, Males and Females, Scientists and Mathematicians' (2001) from the *Journal of Autism and Developmental Disorders*, Vol 31, Issue 1, with permission from Springer Science and Business Media.

Figure 3.5 and **Figure 3.6** are reproduced courtesy of Professor Steven Pinker, Harvard University

Table 5.1 and **Table 5.2** are reproduced courtesy of Professor Simon Baron-Cohen, Autism Research Centre.

Figure 5.1 is reproduced from T Shallice, 'Philosophical Transactions of the Royal Society of London. Series B, Biological Science (1934-1990)' (1985) Volume 298, Number 1089, pp.199-209, with permission from The Royal Society of London.

Figure 5.2 is reproduced with permission of Dr Stephen Karp.

Figure 5.3 is reproduced with permission of Mrs Evelyn Witkin, on behalf of the late Dr Herman A. Witkin.

Figure 5.4 is adapted from the Navon Test of Local-Global Perception.

Figure 5.5 is reproduced courtesy of Professor Simon Baron-Cohen, Cambridge University.

Figure 5.6 is reproduced from Baron-Cohen et al, 'Does the autistic child have a theory of mind?' (1985) from *Cognition,* Volume 21, Issue 1, pp.37-46, with permission of Elsevier.

Figure 5.7 is reproduced from Baron-Cohen et al, 'The "Reading the Mind in the Eyes" Test Revised Version: A Study with Normal Adults, and Adults with Asperger Syndrome or High-Functioning Autism' (2001) from the *Journal of Child Psychology and Psychiatry,* Vol 42, Issue 2, pp.241-251, with permission of Blackwell Publishing.

Figure 5.8 is adapted from the test reported in Baron-Cohen et al, 'Studies of the Theory of Mind: Are intuitive physics and intuitive psychology independent?' (2001) from the *Journal of Developmental and Learning Disorders,* Vol 5, Number 1, pp. 47-80, with permission of the Interdisciplinary Council on Developmental and Learning Disorders.

Figure 5.9 is reproduced from Baron-Cohen et al, 'Studies of the Theory of Mind: Are intuitive physics and intuitive psychology independent?' (2001) from the *Journal of Developmental and Learning Disorders,* Vol 5, Number 1, pp. 47-80, with permission of the Interdisciplinary Council on Developmental and Learning Disorders

Figure 5.10 is reproduced courtesy of Professor Simon Baron-Cohen, Autism Research Centre, Cambridge University.

Table 5.3 and **Figure 5.11** are reproduced from N Goldenfield, S Baron-Cohen, S Wheelwright, 'Empathizing and systemizing in males, females, and autism' (2005) from *Clinical Neuropsychiatry* 2; 338-345, with permission of Giovanni Fioriti, MD, Psychiatrist.

Figure 6.1 is provided with permission of the Magnetic Resonance and Image Analysis Research Centre (MARIARC), University of Liverpool, UK.

Figure 6.2 is adapted from an image supplied courtesy of Dr Chris Ashwin, Autism Research Centre, Cambridge University

Figure 6.3 is reproduced from H Honda et al, 'No effect of MMR withdrawal on the incidence of autism: a total population study' (2005) from the *Journal of Child Psychology and Psychiatry,* Vol 26, Issue 6, pp.572-579 with permission of Blackwell Publishing.

Figure 7.1 is reproduced with kind permission of the photographer, Kate Baron

Figure 7.2 and 7.3 are reproduced with kind permission of Mrs. Anna Maria Perini, on behalf of Lisa Perini.

Figure 7.4 and **Figure 7.5** are reproduced from P Myers, S Baron-Cohen and Sally Wheelwright, 'An Exact Mind: An Artist with Asperger Syndrome' (2004), by permission of Jessica Kingsley Publishers.

Figure 7.6 is reproduced from S Baron-Cohen, O Golan, S Wheelwright, and J Hill, 'Mind Reading (DVD)', (2004), Jessica Kingsley Publishers, courtesy of the Autism Research Centre, Cambridge University.
http://www.jkp.com/mindreading

Figure 7.7 and **Figure 7.8** are reproduced from *The Transporters*, Department for Culture, Media and Sport. © Crown copyright material is reproduced with the permission of the Controller of HMSO and Queen's Printer for Scotland. http://www.thetransporters.com

1

Meeting two people on the autistic spectrum

➡ Key points

Classic autism and Asperger syndrome *share* two key features:

- Social communication difficulties

- Narrow interests and repetitive actions.

But they *differ* in two key ways:

- In Asperger syndrome, IQ is at least average and there was no language delay

- In classic autism, IQ can be anywhere on the scale, and there was language delay.

The quickest way to introduce you to classic autism and Asperger syndrome is to describe a child with each of these diagnoses. Because these conditions change with age, I describe how these two people have turned out as young adults. These individuals are compilations of real people I have met over the years. They are chosen in order to illustrate quite how wide the spectrum is, but also to reveal what it is that individuals on the spectrum all share. It is a sure-fire way to jump straight into the issues of what the autistic spectrum is, and the debate about whether the two major subgroups (of classic autism and Asperger syndrome) should really be 'lumped together' or 'split apart'.

Jamie

Jamie has classic autism (also sometimes called *autistic disorder*). As a child, his favourite activities included bouncing on his trampoline (which he could do for literally hours), flapping a piece of string close to his eyes (which he still does for hours), spinning the wheel of a toy car (which he often engaged in for hours), asking to be swung on his hammock (again, something he could enjoy for hours) or letting sand fall through his fingers. He was also most content when nothing unexpected happened. Unexpected change would trigger a violent tantrum.

Although Jamie is now 19 years old, he has very little speech. He can say parts of words, but these are really only intelligible to his mother and to the small team of carers who help his mother.

All through childhood he slept about 2 hours each night, and otherwise ran up and down in his bedroom, along what almost seemed like an invisible track, so repetitive were his movements. If Jamie wasn't running up and down he would be spinning round and around, as if on a high-speed merry-go-round, but remarkably never experiencing dizziness or losing his balance. He could maintain this circular spinning for hours.

His other unusual bodily movement was his rocking back and forth in a chair. It would start with a gentle rocking and his arms would go back as his head went forward. It would increase in tempo and force until he was rocking like a mechanical metronome, regular as clockwork, and in a trance-like state. This kind of repetitive movement would become faster and faster, growing in intensity, if he was absorbed in a favourite activity, such as watching a DVD that he knew inside out. Jamie wasn't unhappy during these very physical, repetitive activities. Far from it. He would hum, and his hum turned into a rhythmic singing, with a huge smile on his face. The repetition seemed pleasurable until it had reached a climax when he would stop, as suddenly as he had started.

His mother regularly booked herself into a hotel, alone, just to get a good night's sleep, since nights were always broken by Jamie's shouting. Even today, his sleep is patchy, and he is often awake for many hours in the night, ordering and reordering his DVD collection on his shelf, putting his face close to the pages of a model railway catalogue so that he can look at the small print under literally thousands of examples of model trains, thumbing through the well-worn magazine. Often he lies on the carpet, his face on one side, so that he can look at the wheels of his toy train from millimetres away.

Jamie rarely makes eye contact, though sometimes (even with complete strangers) he will put his face very close to theirs, and stare at them in a way that feels uncomfortable for the other person. He frequently still takes off all his clothes, no matter who is visiting or where he is, at home, in the shops or on the bus. This has always been a problem, something his mother has been unable to teach him to inhibit. Sometimes he undoes his flies and starts masturbating, whether at the day centre or with his grandmother, or with one of the young female carers who attempt to restrain him. He shows no embarrassment or social awareness of how others might see him. He started puberty early, at 11, with a faint moustache and sideburns.

He insists on the same food every day, strawberry jam sandwiches, and resists any attempt by his mother to introduce more variety into his diet. He frequently goes for 2 weeks without a bowel movement, and has suffered all his life with the pain of gastrointestinal blockages. His mother heaves an audible sigh of relief when he passes a motion, since this signals a few days of calmer behaviour on Jamie's part.

He insists on wearing the same brown corduroy trousers, summer or winter, and the same hand-knitted sweater. Jamie also wears a sun hat, day and night, refusing to take it off even to sleep. If his mother wants to wash his trousers or sweater, she has to do this in the evening, because he will not wear any other clothes in the day. She has never managed to wash the sun hat that by now is worn and misshapen, and for a quiet life she lets him wear it. Sometimes he appears frustrated and bites the back of his hand, drawing blood.

He still walks in a very distinct way, not swinging his arms, while leaning forward on tip toe. He always chooses to walk on the inside of the pavement, and his hand trails along the walls of the buildings, touching them ever so lightly, as he avoids people and glides through the city.

His mother is tireless in her care of him, but occasionally Jamie hugs her too tight and she has to push him away because of his physical strength. As a child, left to his own devices, he would find his favourite videotape of *Thomas The Tank Engine*, put it into the VCR, use the remote to fast-forward to a particular scene where a carriage becomes separated from the train pulling it, and rewind and play and rewind and play that brief sequence over and over again. His mother tried to replace the videotape but Jamie insisted on the original version of the tape, despite the fact that the tape was worn away in places, and had crackles and hisses in different places. Jamie could echo or imitate these crackles and hisses, in the correct sequence and with exact timing, even though he has little spontaneous speech. He also mimicked the narrator on the tape, producing the words with precise intonation and timing.

Suddenly, at the age of 12, after years of watching *Thomas The Tank Engine* every day, Jamie latched onto a new videotape of the *Severn Valley Railway* and that became the tape he then wanted to watch over and over again.

Despite his lack of useful language, his hearing is clearly excellent, as he can not only imitate the sounds of the trains with exactness, but gets upset if the kitchen clock is ticking, asking his mother to remove the battery. His vision is also excellent, in that even though he hardly reads books, he can recognize a model number in a catalogue even if it is across the room. If you ask Jamie to call out the number you are pointing at, from the other side of the room, he can read it accurately.

When he is not watching his video, which he does for many hours a day, he will walk around the room, tapping the surfaces of the walls, furniture, windows or objects in the room, as if to confirm the feel of the textures and the sound of the tapping, his movements producing the same sound over and over again. Efforts to engage him in play or conversation or emotional exchange, or even a joint activity lead nowhere. He will look past the other person, as if totally preoccupied by his own thoughts. When he wants something, he will take their hand and place it on the object, or if the object is out of reach, take their hand and throw it towards the object, all the while not making any eye contact and treating the hand as if it was disconnected from its owner.

On a crowded beach, if Jamie spots something he wants, he will have no hesitation to make a bee-line for the object, even if it means stepping over or even on the sunbathers. Once, in a kitchen showroom in the local shopping arcade, he spotted a demonstration toilet on display. Before his mother had realized what he had done, he had climbed onto the toilet and defecated. His mother was alerted by the store assistant because Jamie was staring into the toilet bowl and starting to rock backwards and forwards. She spends much of their time in public explaining in embarrassed tones that he has autism, and her levels of stress are high. Not infrequently he runs away, and often is found back at home, having found his way home from anywhere in the city, by following the bus routes.

Jamie was diagnosed at the age of 4 years old with classic autism. Some of his behaviour when he was young was just dismissed as cute or child-like, socially naïve, but seeing the same behaviours in a tall teenager makes them stand out as atypical. He has grabbed his mother's hot cup of tea, freshly poured from the boiling kettle, and drunk all of the boiling tea without pausing for a breath, with no apparent pain. Whilst his constipation can leave him crying in pain, at other times (after a fall and a cut or a bump) he will carry on 'twiddling' his piece of string near his eyes, without communicating any pain or indicating that he has an injury.

He attended a special school for 'low-functioning' children with autism, where the educational method was 'Applied Behavioural Analysis' (ABA).

There were six children in each class, with two classroom assistants in addition to the class teacher. Jamie paid no attention to the other children in the class, except one boy who wore glasses. Jamie liked to grab this boy's glasses and throw them across the room, something the teacher or classroom assistants had to be alert to at all times. If Jamie succeeded, he laughed out loud, even if he was reprimanded or put into the time-out corner of the room.

Apart from his diagnosis of autism, he is also diagnosed as having learning difficulties. This is because although he is 19, his skills on standardized tests of intelligence score in the range of a 12 year old or younger.

Jamie has one older sister, Alice, who is shy, withdrawn and obsessed with the band *Red Hot Chili Peppers*. She has spent all her savings on memorabilia related to this band, and her bedroom walls, shelves and window sill are crammed full of posters, concert programmes, CDs and pop magazines related to this band. She dresses in black only, with heavy black mascara, and reads deeply in the topic of green politics. She is very judgmental of anyone who does not agree with her view of the world. She describes herself as having some autistic traits.

Jamie's parents divorced when Jamie was 12. They attribute the stress of looking after Jamie as a major cause of their marital difficulties. Jamie's father has remarried and his new partner, Georgia, is expecting a baby. Georgia is quite worried about whether the new baby might develop autism too. Jamie's mother remains single, and is on long-term antidepressants, as the periods when she has tried to live without them have left her at times suicidal. But she knows that Jamie depends so much on her that she has to find the will to live, for him.

Jamie's case illustrates the impact of autism on both him and his family. Having met a person with classic autism, we now need to meet Andrew, who has received a diagnosis in the other major subgroup on the autistic spectrum, Asperger syndrome.

Andrew

Andrew is also 19 years old. He has always had remarkably advanced language. He was speaking his first words at 9 months and by 18 months he had a precocious vocabulary. His very first word was in fact a two-word phrase: 'articulated lorry'. His parents were very proud and told visitors about their extraordinary, advanced child. By 2 years old he was reading the small print on the back of all the video cases in the family collection, and by 5 he could name which censorship code each one had received (12, or 15, or Adult Viewing), for thousands of videos in the local video store. By 3, he would accompany his father to the video store and run up and down the aisles, putting videos back in their correct place when other customers had sloppily misclassified them.

Andrew would also look along any skirting board of any room he was in, scanning for electrical outlets, and if there was no appliance plugged in, he would flick the switch to the off position. By 4 he had started collecting football stickers and could name every picture of any footballer in the Premiere League, and give their statistics (goal average, which teams he had played for, when he joined the present club, what price the club paid for him, etc.).

Andrew was never interested in talking to other children his own age, and instead gravitated towards adults who he talked at, rather than with. He would tell anyone who listened all the details of the *Harry Potter* novels, and would talk about the novels for hours if not interrupted. He didn't need any reply to his monologue. He spent hours in his bedroom alone, happy to make lists of his favourite songs or his favourite films, or his favourite cars, or his favourite Harry Potter spells. His mother sometimes joked that Andrew made so many lists that he needed lists of all his lists!

Andrew was frequently in trouble at primary school for ignoring the timetable, instead reading an encyclopedia that he carried around with him, or arranging all the cut grass in the field behind the school into neat, straight lines. Often he would shout out in class the words 'Why?' or 'How do you know?' whenever the teacher made an assertion of fact. The teacher felt in a dilemma. She could see that Andrew had a natural curiosity that she didn't want to stifle. On the other hand, she found it was very disruptive to the other pupils and was frustrated that Andrew did not seem to be able to conform to the social norms of not interrupting, or joining in group activities. When Andrew was reprimanded for constantly interrupting he protested that if a teacher or indeed anyone says something that is not factually correct then they were 'wrong', 'talking rubbish' and were 'telling lies'. Andrew felt he had a duty to tell the truth and to point out when information was incorrect. His nick-name became error-checker.

Andrew would also annoy the teachers because he wanted to go into far more depth in any given topic than they could cover or even knew. For example, at 14 years old, when studying the history of the Second World War, Andrew became interested in the Battle of Monte Cassino, which began on the 4th January 1944. Whilst the rest of the class had finished History and had moved on to French, Andrew was still interested in the small details of that one battle: how many soldiers had died, what their names were, what dates each had died, how and where each had been killed, how many had survived, the names of the survivors, their ranks, their uniforms, the insignia on their uniforms, the route they had taken, where they were marching, etc.

He saw no reason to stop reading about the one battle, since to claim you had learnt about that battle in history was simply a lie if there were facts that had not been unearthed and covered. His mind was driven to go to the ultimate end of a topic, until there was no new information available. At that point, he was ready to move to a new topic. It annoyed him that the teacher and the other children said the Battle of Monte Cassino had become his 'preoccupation', or that he was 'obsessed'. For him, if a subject was worth learning, it was worth learning properly, or not at all. He was shocked at what passed for education in his class, which seemed to him such a superficial, vague, broad-brush sketch of a topic that it was next to worthless. He described most people he met as stupid, and had little respect for people who could not answer questions of fact with precision. Nor could he understand the concept of 'human error' when other people recalled information inaccurately.

Occasionally an adult friend of his parents who had an area of expertise (such as wine-making, or Russian language) would visit his home and he would enjoy asking them lots of questions about their specialist area of knowledge. The adult would feel pinned to the wall by Andrew's barrage of questions, commenting that it was like an interrogation, as if Andrew was trying to download knowledge from their mind to his. Sometimes the questioning would start in the most inappropriate place, such as when they had just entered the front door and were still in the hallway, not having seen Andrew for several years. Andrew seemed to have little sense of what was socially appropriate, when enough was enough, or when he might be being intrusive or even boring.

When he was 7 or 8, other children would tease Andrew in the playground. Once they even put him in the school dustbin. He learned to be fearless in fighting back and got into trouble for violence, even though he is adamant that he never starts conflict. He became fascinated by numbers at age 12 and took his GCSE maths exam 4 years earlier than is normal, obtaining an A* grade. (This is an exam usually taken at age 16). This was the only national exam he took, because he thought the History syllabus was designed for idiots, that the science books didn't look at *how* things worked, but just got you to label diagrams of parts of the eye or list the properties of living things. He wanted to know *how* a cell actually worked, since for him it was no different from the kitchen toaster he had taken apart and reassembled. It was a small, beautiful machine.

English lessons he found a total waste of time, because the teacher asked unanswerable questions such as 'What do you think the author was feeling?' or 'What is the significance of the dream sequence in *Death of a Salesman*?' He asked his head teacher if he could just drop all other subjects except maths because maths was logical, precise, and each new fact or rule built on a previous one.

He loved patterns in maths and his favourite number was the Golden Ratio of 1.6180339887.

The head teacher said that she was required by UK law to ensure that all children covered the National Curriculum, which included all the subjects he wanted to drop. Andrew laughed in her face, telling her that she was running an institution where children learnt a little about lots of things and almost nothing about a single topic. He accused her of being anti-education. She told him that was the law. He argued back that education was about knowledge, and knowledge was about understanding how details fit together, or why things are the way they are, be they natural phenomena like the chemistry causing the colours in a rock, or be they human events, like how many votes each candidate got in each constituency which led to the Prime Minister's election. He shouted that he was not interested in learning 10 facts about the Second World War to pass an exam. He picked up her globe on her desk, told her it offended him because the country boundaries had all changed since that globe had been made so it was not correct, and threw it through a closed window. He was excluded for 1 week.

Because the bullying did not stop, Andrew lost motivation in going into school and dropped out of school by age 15. At 18, having spent 3 years at home, he taught himself every song written for guitar in the 1970s (his favourite era) and created his own language, called *Origenish*, which he said was the original human language, each word being a mix of Hindi and Hebrew, with its own dictionary and grammar book. He still believed everyone else was more stupid than him, but this arrogant attitude seemed to be contradicted by his lack of school qualifications. He decided to teach himself some A levels, and obtained six A levels in 1 year (three in arts subjects and three in sciences).

On the strength of these results, he returned to education by applying to university, to study Natural Sciences. He has learnt the names of every protein and can describe their 3D structure. He still makes lists, but confesses he has no idea how to have a conversation and would not dream of going into a pub. His biggest fear is 'small talk', which he says is totally beyond him. At university, he saw a poster on a notice board about Asperger syndrome, and realized this must apply to him. He took himself off to the local clinic and the diagnosis was confirmed. When he received his diagnosis, he stood up and shook the hand of the doctor, much to the amazement of his parents who had come along to the assessment. He finally felt he belonged and that he had a name for why he had always felt different from everyone. He just wished he could have had his diagnosis in childhood, to have got the proper recognition that his learning style was different, to be recognized as a vulnerable target for the school bullies, and he regretted the 'lost years'.

Andrew went on to the Internet and discovered lots of people with Asperger syndrome, who he now regularly e-mails and even meets up with to go to events such as the re-enactment of the Battle of Monte Cassino. He describes the minds of other people, so-called 'neurotypicals', as like butterflies: hopping from topic to topic with no linearity. He cannot see the point of neurotypical conversation. He enjoys talking to someone only to get information or to provide information, or to prove a point of fact. He readily admits he has no diplomacy skills, since he always just says what he thinks. He cannot understand the need to 'sugar the pill', and finds metaphors puzzling. He admits he has no real friends though he considers the cleaner who tidies his room and the woman in the supermarket his friends because they say hello to him every day. Sometimes he suffers from clinical depression.

Andrew avoids change totally. He always goes to bed at 3 am, describing himself as nocturnal. He eats away from the rest of the family, in his bedroom. He sits at his computer, solving maths problems, in the dark. If his mother comes in and turns on the lights or opens the curtains, he totally loses his train of thought and can become angry with her, even throwing things. He always eats the same food every day: digestive biscuits and milk. He defends his diet as providing everything he needs for his health and as very economic. He doesn't care what others think of his odd tastes, as the only views that count are his own.

Every 15 minutes he checks the weather forecast on the radio and writes down the latest report in a little notebook, with neat columns for the temperature, rainfall, wind speed and humidity. He still watches his favourite films over and over again, and says that some of them he has watched several hundred times. He finds the noise of a fly in the room painfully loud and refuses to go in there unless the fly is removed.

Sometimes he feels like he is from a different planet, from Mars, because he cannot understand or participate in the things that other people seem to do easily. Things that are so ordinary to other people, such as reading their faces, knowing what to say next in a conversation, knowing how to comfort some-one, knowing what not to say to avoid upsetting someone or simply getting a joke. He has had this sense of being a Martian ever since school days, when he could see the other children playing games in the playground that didn't have clear rules. He had no idea how they knew what to do. He still talks *at* people rather than *to* them. On one occasion whilst on the phone he carried on talk-ing for 10 minutes after the phone had gone dead, not realizing no-one was listening at the other end.

Whilst Andrew can do maths, or memorize facts, or understand the laws of chemistry or physics effortlessly, he cannot fathom the unspoken rules of human interaction. He has at times felt suicidal but continues to take hope from other people with Asperger syndrome whom he has met via the web, who all feel the same, and who are struggling with the same feelings: of marginalization, alienated on a planet where they do not feel they belong. The growing recognition of Asperger syndrome being neurologically 'atypical' rather than 'disordered' is one he finds more respectful of how he is different. He often likens Asperger syndrome to being left-handed, in the days when to be left-handed was to be regarded as 'sinister' and in need of treatment. Nowadays he is comforted by the idea that a percentage of the population will develop differently, as a result of their different wiring in the brain.

What do Jamie and Andrew share?

Jamie has classic autism and Andrew has Asperger syndrome (a term I prefer over the official term Asperger Disorder). They both share the core diagnostic features: difficulties in social development, and in the development of communication, alongside unusually strong, narrow interests and repetitive behaviour. These diagnostic features are enshrined in the *Diagnostic and Statistical Manual* (DSM), now in its fourth edition (DSM-IV), produced by the American Psychiatric Association. They are also enshrined in the European equivalent, the *International Classification of Diseases* (ICD), now in its 10th edition (ICD-10), produced by the World Health Organization.

These diagnostic features are sometimes referred to as the 'triad' of autism, because they comprise three key areas of atypical development (for short: social, communication and repetition). I don't think one can separate the social and communication domains (since communication is always social). It might be more fruitful to think of autism and Asperger syndrome as sharing features in two broad areas: social communication and narrow interests/ repetitive actions.

It is because individuals with classic autism or Asperger syndrome share these features that they are lumped together. Classification in science has always debated whether two things should be lumped together or split apart. Scientists fluctuate as to whether to side with the lumpers or the splitters. Those who lump classic autism and Asperger syndrome together argue that in the long run this will be more fruitful because they are both the same kind of condition, lying on the same underlying *autistic spectrum*. Those who argue for splitting them apart argue that their differences are greater than their similarities.

Given that in classic autism the person may also have learning difficulties and language delay, it is sometimes said that classic autism is much more severe than Asperger syndrome. Certainly, the presence of learning difficulties is bound to limit the individual's potential, both academically and occupationally, as well as their self-help and independence skills. There is no easy way to measure 'severity' though, since if a person is suffering because of gastrointestinal pain (common in classic autism) or depression (common in Asperger syndrome), both can be 'severe'. If you are the person with one of these conditions, and if it is causing you to suffer in some way, even if simply interfering with your ability to do ordinary things such as making friends, that can feel 'severe'. But if one takes a view from the outside, rather than in terms of 'how it feels', one could say that classic autism is likely to lead to *more* disabilities than Asperger syndrome.

If we are lumping these two subgroups together, it is because they both fall in the intersection of the Venn diagram in Figure 1.1. This also helps us understand why both subgroups fall on the same autistic spectrum. They share the cluster of features. A person who had just a single feature (social communication difficulties, or just narrow interests) would not end up with a diagnosis on the autistic spectrum. But a person who showed both features would.

How do Jamie and Andrew differ?

Whereas Jamie was late to talk and never developed mature speech, Andrew talked early and his vocabulary was precocious. So age of onset of speech production and language comprehension is the first big difference between classic autism and Asperger syndrome. Indeed, the diagnosis of Asperger syndrome requires that the child spoke on time. This requirement is not the case for a diagnosis of classic autism.

Secondly, Jamie has obvious learning difficulties, such that he had to attend a special school and never completed national exams in academic subjects. On an IQ test his scores are well below average. The average (or mean) on an IQ test is 100, and the range is two 'standard deviations' (SDs) from the mean (where 1 SD is 15 points). So a person with an IQ as low as 70 would still be considered within the average range.

Jamie is currently 19 years old but is considered to have a 'mental age' of an 11 year old. If you take a young person's mental age and divide this by their chronological age, multiplied by 100, you get their IQ. So his IQ can be calculated

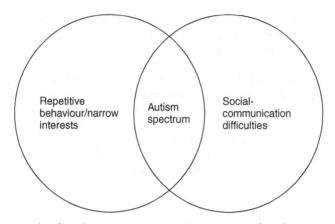

Figure 1.1 Identifying the autistic spectrum as the intersection of two features, i.e., those individuals who show both features.

as $(11/19) \times 100 = 58$. This is clearly in the below-average range. In contrast, Andrew is gifted in certain areas (e.g. maths), and has ended up in university. A good rule of thumb is that to get to university one is likely to have an IQ more than 1 SD above the mean (i.e. an IQ of at least 115). So, IQ is the second major difference between classic autism and Asperger syndrome. Indeed, the diagnosis of Asperger syndrome requires that the child has average IQ or above. This requirement is not the case for a diagnosis of classic autism.

Terminology

The differences between classic autism and Asperger syndrome are shown visually in Figure 1.2.

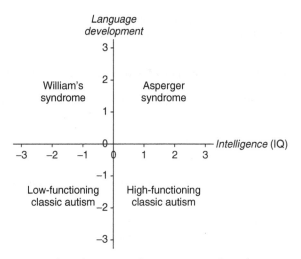

Figure 1.2 Distinguishing classic autism from Asperger syndrome.[1]

To reiterate, classic autism and Asperger syndrome both share two key features:

- Social communication difficulties.

- Narrow interests and repetitive actions.

But classic autism and Asperger syndrome differ in two key ways:

- In Asperger syndrome, IQ is at least average and there was no language delay.

- In classic autism, IQ can be anywhere on the scale, and there was language delay.

The definition of what counts as language delay is quite clear-cut. If the child is not producing single words by the age of 2, or phrase speech by the age of 3, then they are defined as delayed in language.

The definition of what counts as average IQ is a little more contentious. Most clinicians would say that this needs to be above 70, as this is 2 SDs below the mean. My own view is that IQ needs to be above 85 (which is 1 SD below the mean) in order to be conservative in one's definition of 'average'. This is because an IQ as low as 70 does carry with it significant educational challenges.

It may be helpful to think of there being six major subgroups on the autistic spectrum, who all have the two key features listed above:

- *Asperger syndrome* (IQ is above 85 and there was no language delay).

- *High-functioning autism* (IQ is above 85 and there was language delay).

- *Medium-functioning autism* (IQ is 71–84 with or without language delay).

- *Low-functioning autism* (IQ is less than 70 with or without language delay).

- *Atypical autism* (either atypical *late* onset or atypical because of having only one rather than two of the core features).

- *Pervasive developmental disorder—not otherwise specified* (where the features are too mild to warrant a clear-cut diagnosis of autism or Asperger syndrome, but where the individual has more than the usual number of autistic traits [2]).

Autism spectrum disorder (ASD) versus autism spectrum condition (ASC)

The official terminology is to use the acronym ASD, for autism spectrum disorder. I prefer the acronym ASC, since individuals in the high-functioning subgroup are certainly different—they think differently and perceive differently—but it is arguable whether these differences should be seen as a *disorder*. Certainly, whilst social skills in people with ASC are invariably below average (by definition), non-social skills (e.g., attention to detail) are often above average. This profile of strengths and difficulties is described in Chapter 4.

The term *condition* I think is a convenient way of recognizing that for individuals or their families who find their way to a clinic—presumably because these features are causing problems and they are seeking help— this profile requires a medical diagnosis, because this profile arises from neurobiological factors (described in Chapter 5). The term 'condition' simultaneously acknowledges the disabling aspects of autism and Asperger syndrome, and the fact that the differences in functioning do not lead to *global* disability, and may in some individuals even result in talent.

2

The changing prevalence of autism through history

> ### ➲ Key points
>
> ◦ 30 years ago, autism was rare (4 in 10,000). Today it is common (1 in 100).
>
> ◦ The categorical view of autism has been replaced by the spectrum view. A direct consequence of this has been to open the clinic door to the 'milder' cases of autism spectrum conditions who also needed to be recognized because they were suffering in childhood, and who were either not diagnosed at all, or who were perhaps diagnosed in other ways.
>
> ◦ It is a welcome development that increased diagnosis, mostly due to better recognition, means more people potentially may now get their special needs met.
>
> ◦ Although the world is beginning to become more autism-friendly, many individuals and their families continue to suffer through insufficient support.

Autism as a 'categorically distinct disorder'

If you went back to 1978, the prevailing view was that autism was categorical: you either have it or you don't. Child psychiatrist Michael Rutter (Figure 2.1), (working at London's Institute of Psychiatry) cited the rate of autism as 4 children in every 10 000, a figure based on a prevalence study by Victor Lotter. Rutter made a major contribution to the classification and recognition of autism by distinguishing it from other psychiatric conditions (e.g., childhood

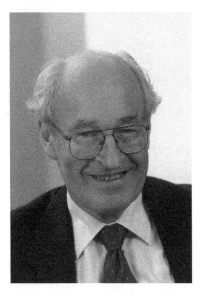

Figure 2.1 Professor Sir Michael Rutter, MD, whose work helped to draw attention to autism as a medical condition, and who first discovered evidence for genetic factors in autism.

schizophrenia), other developmental conditions (e.g., specific language impairment), and by clarifying the diagnostic criteria.

Classic autism is also sometimes called 'Kanner's autism' after Leo Kanner (Figure 2.2), the child psychiatrist who had first described these children in 1943. He recognized 11 children in his clinic in Baltimore who had what he called 'autistic aloneness', showing so little interest in people that they may as well have been furniture in his office. He borrowed the word 'autism' from its use by the Swiss psychiatrist Bleuler, who had used it to describe schizophrenia. The word autism comes from the Greek word 'autos' that literally means 'self'. It was a well-chosen word, because autism and Asperger syndrome involve a profound difficulty in appreciating another person's different perspective, as if one's own perspective were the true, correct view.

In Chapter 1 we listed two main diagnostic areas (social communication difficulties, and narrow interests/repetitive behaviour). From Kanner's and Rutter's descriptions, we can break these down into specific behaviours.

Social difficulties

- Extreme lack of interest in other people.

- Atypical eye contact: either hardly making eye contact, or staring at you for too long, invading your personal space.

- Lack of reciprocity (no turn-taking, no dialogue, just monologue).

- Preferring to be alone.

- Difficulties anticipating how someone will feel or what they might think.

- Difficulties knowing how to react to another person's behaviour.

- Difficulty reading other people's emotional expressions, in their face or voice or posture.

- Difficulty accepting that there may be other perspectives, not just a single correct perspective.

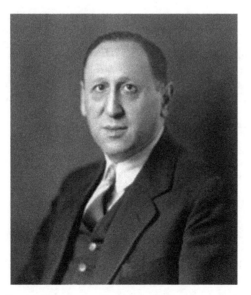

Figure 2.2 Leo Kanner, MD, who first described what we now recognize as classic autism.

Communication abnormalities

- Echolalic speech (echoing phrases*).

- Neologisms (using idiosyncratic words instead of conventional names for things*).

- Literal understanding of speech.

- Language delay to varying degrees*.

- Using speech inappropriately for the social context (pragmatics abnormalities).

Repetitive behaviour and narrow interests

- Hand-flapping*.

- Spinning of the body*.

- Obsessional interests (e.g. touching everything, collecting stones, collecting ladybirds, collecting information on a narrow topic, etc.).

- Lining things up.

- Spinning the wheels of a toy car, and becoming mesmerized by spinning objects (e.g. washing machines, blades of fans, windmills).

- Highly repetitive behaviour.

- Severe tantrums at change.

- Splinter skills or islets of intelligence.

- Unusual memory.

- Need for sameness.

(*More typical of classic autism than Asperger syndrome).

Other features that do not clearly fall into the above categories

- Areas of below-average IQ or learning difficulties*.

- High risk of epilepsy*.

- Self-injury*.

- Hypersensitivity to sounds, textures, tastes, smells, temperature.

(*More typical of classic autism than Asperger syndrome).

Chicago-based psychoanalyst Bruno Bettelheim (Figure 2.3) in the 1960s portrayed children with autism as living 'in a glass bubble', unreachable. He viewed autism as a reaction to an unaffectionate maternal relationship. Bettelheim's controversial view led to a form of treatment called 'parentectomy', or removal of the child from his or her parents, in the hope that the child's social development would recover and blossom with foster parents who could be affectionate.

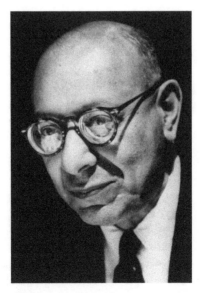

Figure 2.3 Bruno Bettelheim, whose theory of autism as a reaction to inadequate parenting has been disproved.

His ideas and his treatment methods fell into disrepute when it was recognized that removal of the child from the biological parents did not lead to an obvious improvement in the child's social development, and when it was recognized (following Michael Rutter's important studies of families) that parents of children with autism were no less caring than other parents. Thanks to Rutter's seminal scientific contributions, parents were no longer to blame for their child's unusual behaviour. Sadly it has taken decades for some parents to feel really free of the guilt that Bettelheim's theory implied.

Nobel Prize-winning ethologist Niko Tinbergen (Figure 2.4), based in Oxford, reinforced Bettelheim's view in his 1983 book, when he speculated that any emotional trauma that disrupts the child's primary attachment to their mother (including brief separations on a long car journey for a particularly anxious child) could cause autism. Whilst Tinbergen should be acknowledged for having highlighted the high levels of social anxiety that many children with autism show, again there was no evidence for his view that the autism itself arose following a trauma of some kind. Moreover, the controversial treatment he

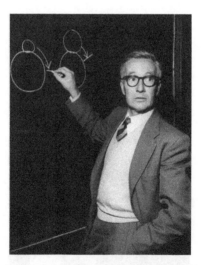

Figure 2.4 Professor Niko Tinbergen, whose Nobel Prize was for his work in the field of ethology (animal behaviour) but whose Nobel Prize acceptance speech speculated about autism being the result of psychological trauma. This theory is no longer tenable.

endorsed, called *Holding Therapy* (or forced hugging, to break through the child's aversion to being touched or held), has been questioned on ethical grounds, given that often the child finds it very distressing to be forced into social contact in this way.

Although Rutter's research had thankfully shown that autism was not due to cold mothering, the image of the unreachable child, together with the core feature of *social unrelatedness*, fostered all sorts of fantasies about these children: that they were similar to feral children, foundlings, evolutionary throwbacks, missing links, even from another planet. All of these views were mythical, and the subsequent decades of research established that autism is a neurological condition.

In the period from 1943 to the late 1980s, children with classic autism were largely seen as distinct from the rest of the population, with a rare, severe *disorder*. This is shown in Figure 2.5. Between the two groups of children was clear blue water. There was no grey zone.

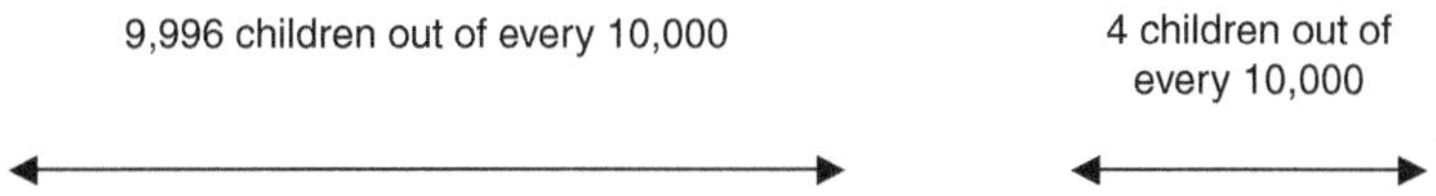

9,996 children out of every 10,000   4 children out of
every 10,000

Figure 2.5 Autism as rare and categorically distinct.

Autism as a spectrum condition

Dr Lorna Wing is a social psychiatrist, parent of a daughter (Suzie) with classic autism, and one of the founding parents of the National Autistic Society (NAS). She worked in the Medical Research Council's (MRC) Social Psychiatry Unit in London. She conducted a prevalence study based on the population with learning disabilities (in those days called 'mental handicap'). She argued that autism lay on a *spectrum*, that it was not categorical, and that if you took the spectrum view, the prevalence of autism was 10–20 per 10 000 (or 1–2 per 1000).

So, whilst the prevailing view was that autism was a rare, categorical disorder, Lorna Wing (Figure 2.6) suggested that autism was a spectrum condition affecting as many as 1 in 500 children with IQ's less than 70 (i.e., just classic autism).

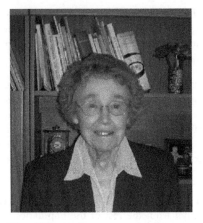

Figure 2.6 Dr. Lorna Wing, MD, who first suggested autism was a spectrum of conditions and that autism may be much more common.

Hans Asperger (Figure 2.7) had picked out a different kind of child, with different features that included the following:

- No language delay.

- Pedantic style of speech.

- Precocious vocabulary development.

- Narrow interests (e.g. flags of the world, weather maps, the history of the railway, etc.).

- A preference for adult company over that of a peer group.

- Bossy and controlling.

- Social oddities that might appear either as social withdrawal or as social intrusiveness.

- A desire for things to be done in the same way over and over again.

- An excellent attention to and memory for detail.

- An IQ in the average range, or above.

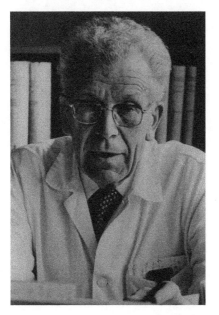

Figure 2.7 Professor Hans Asperger, MD, who first described a high-functioning group of children with autism.

As mentioned in the Introduction, Lorna Wing brought Asperger's ideas to the English-speaking world in 1981, in her article in *Psychological Medicine*, since Asperger had published in his native German whilst working in Austria in 1944. The international committees that decide on diagnostic practice finally recognized this subgroup in 1994.

In Sweden, child psychiatrist Christopher Gillberg (Figure 2.8) found a rate of one child in every 330 had Asperger Syndrome, in 1993. By 2001, a Cambridge study reported rates of one child in every 166 having an autism spectrum condition in a primary school population, and a similar rate (1 in 150) was reported across the Atlantic in the Brick Township. In 2006 paediatrician Gillian Baird (Figure 2.9), working in London at Guy's Hospital, reported in the *Lancet* that 1 per cent of the population met the criteria for an autism spectrum condition.

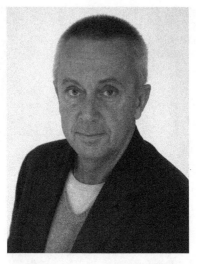

Figure 2.8 Professor Christopher Gillberg, MD, who conducted the first prevalence study of Asperger Syndrome in childhood.

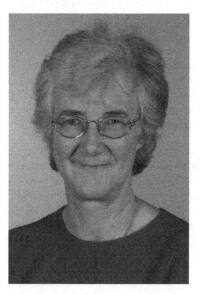

Figure 2.9 Dr. Gillian Baird, MD, who led the team studying the prevalence of ASC in the south-east of England, reporting rates of 1%.

So, by 1990, the situation could be depicted as in Figure 2.10.

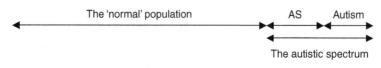

The 'normal' population   AS   Autism

The autistic spectrum

Figure 2.10 The autistic spectrum 'outside' the general population.
(AS = Asperger syndrome.)

By the mid-1990s, two other subgroups were added to the autistic spectrum (Figure 2.11): *atypical autism* (where the features are only partially seen) and *PDD-NOS* (pervasive developmental disorder—not otherwise specified) (where the severity may be of a milder degree).

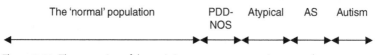

The 'normal' population   PDD-NOS   Atypical   AS   Autism

Figure 2.11 The expansion of the autistic spectrum to recognize new subgroups.
(AS = Asperger syndrome; PDD-NOS = pervasive developmental disorder—not otherwise specified.)

This brief history teaches us two things. First, autism prevalence is not set in stone. In just two decades, it jumped from 4 in 10 000 to 1 per cent, which represents a 25-fold increase. This is shown in Figure 2.12. From what has been said so far, much of this increase reflects the following:

◈ *The shift from categorical to spectrum views of autism.* Now that we recognize shades of autism, we can include not just the extreme cases but also the milder cases.

◈ *Better recognition, better training and better services.* Now that most primary health professionals (e.g., speech therapists, GPs, health visitors, child psychologists, child psychiatrists, paediatricians) are taught about the autistic spectrum and there are clinics to assess it in every small town, not just the big cities, clinics see many more children for assessments than ever before.

◈ *The inclusion of new subgroups.* In the old days only classic autism was recognized, but now children and adults with different forms of autism spectrum condition (Asperger syndrome, atypical autism, PDD-NOS) are included.

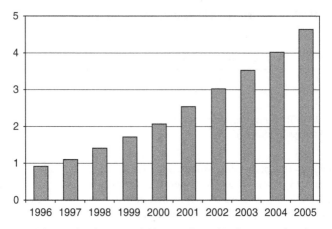

Figure 2.12 The number (per 1000 children aged 6–11) in the USA with a diagnosis of Autism, from 1996 to 2005. This striking graph was put together by someone on the internet who calls him or herself Eubulides. The counts of children diagnosed with autism were taken from Table 1–9 of IDEA Part B Child Count (2005). These were divided by census estimates for the US resident population aged 6–11, taken from US census estimates for 1990–1999 resident population by age and the similar estimates for 2000–2005. Eubulides notes that for all years, the September population estimates were used. [As with anything which has not been peer reviewed, one needs to take this information with a pinch of salt. But there is no real dispute over the fact that the rate of diagnosis of autism spectrum conditions has massively increased.]
See http://en.wikipedia.org/wiki/Autism

Controversies regarding prevalence

There are some controversial new claims that the massive increase in prevalence may reflect other factors, both environmental and genetic. For example, one lobbying group in the USA continues to argue that the MMR (measles, mumps and rubella) vaccination causes autism and is responsible for the increase in rates of the condition. We will return to this in Chapter 6. Suffice it to say that there is no strong evidence either for MMR being a cause of autism, or for it causing the increase in prevalence.

Another lobbying group claims it is not the viruses in the vaccine itself, but the *mercury* base of other childhood vaccines, with suggestions of heavy metal (mercury) toxicity in the brains of children with autism. Specifically, this group claims that children with autism have a genetic inability to *secrete* the mercury that we are all exposed to, with the result that this is carried by the blood, into the brain, and accumulates there. One strand of evidence for their claim is that the amount of mercury found in the hair of children with autism is allegedly *lower* than in comparison groups. This is taken as indirect evidence that it is not being secreted from the brain through the scalp and into the hair, so it must be building up in the brain. This study has been criticized on the grounds that the control group had well below normal levels of mercury in their hair, raising questions not about the autism group, but about how typical the comparison group were.

A more genetic explanation of the increase in prevalence is the idea that parents who are carrying the genes for autism may be more likely to meet each other and start a family than in previous generations. This assumes that autism is primarily genetic (a fact that is no longer in any doubt, as we shall see in Chapter 6), and that both parents contribute 'risk' genes. This is called the 'assortative mating' theory, meaning 'like marries like'. According to this theory, parents of children who have autism may not have autism itself, but may have talents associated with the condition. Thus, children with autism have superior attention to detail in terms of their perception and memory, and they are strongly attracted to systems of different kinds (discussed in Chapter 5). These systems might be collecting objects within a category (toy trains) or mathematical patterns, or train timetables or weather forecasts, as examples. Their parents might have similar characteristics (excellent attention to detail, and a strong interest in systems) and may have even used these in their occupations quite successfully. Famous examples include Jim and Marian Simons, who have a child with autism. Jim and Marian are both mathematics graduates from MIT, and Jim set up one of the world's most successful hedge funds which is today valued at US$1.8 billion. His philanthropic foundation now funds, among other worthy causes, autism research.

Claims in *Wired Magazine* in December 2001 reported that autism was more common in Silicon Valley in California, a place where those with remarkable talents at 'systemizing' might travel to live and work, and where they might meet a partner and start a family. It remains unclear if such assortative mating is operating in autism, or if it plays any part in the rising rates of autism. Some evidence in support of the assortative mating theory is that fathers of children with autism are more likely to be working in the field of engineering (for which you would need good systemizing skills), and that this was also true of their grandfathers on both sides of the family.

Anecdotal reports are that whilst the rate of autism is about 1 per cent in most populations, in Silicon Valley it may be about 10 per cent. If confirmed, this would be strong evidence consistent with the assortative mating theory. Sceptics of this theory argue that genetic change does not happen quickly (over decades) but has a much longer timescale (millions of years). However, there are other medical conditions whose rates have changed within a generation as a result of changes in mating patterns. But we should be cautious about concluding that assortative mating has anything to do with rising rates of autism, pending further evidence, and in the meantime assume that the rising rates mostly reflect more ordinary factors, such as better recognition and the broadening of the category of autism.

3

Measuring the autistic spectrum

➜ Key Points

- The Autism Spectrum Quotient (AQ) is a screening instrument that can be used from 4 years of age through to adulthood. It measures how many autistic traits an individual shows, and can be used right across the population, not just in clinics. The AQ has been tested in terms of its clinical validity. The AQ still needs to be evaluated for its utililty as a population screen. This will entail evaluating what proportion of cases in a population the instrument correctly detects.

- There are related versions for children (the Child AQ) or teenagers (the Adolescent AQ). There is also a toddler version, the Q-CHAT (Quantitative Checklist for Autism in Todlers). [These are all freely available as downloadable files at www.autismresearchcentre.com.]

- If you are a parent or a professional and are concerned about whether a particular child or adult might have an autism spectrum condition (ASC), the AQ can be a quick, useful indicator to determine if a full diagnostic assessment is warranted. Adults who are high-functioning and who suspect they might have ASC can also fill in the AQ themselves, for the same purpose.

- A high AQ score alone is not a reason to be referred for a diagnosis. In addition, there has to also be evidence that the person is 'suffering' in some way (e.g. they are being bullied, or are becoming depressed, or have high levels of anxiety, or are not fulfilling their academic or occupational potential). A referral to a specialist clinic is then warranted. The diagnostic assessment needs to be conducted by a trained clinician (a psychiatrist, a paediatrician or a clinical psychologist, for example), usually through a direct interview with an informant who knew the 'patient' as a young child.

Today the notion of an autistic spectrum is no longer defined by any sharp separation from 'normality'. The clearest way of seeing this 'normal' distribution of autistic traits is by looking at the results from the *Autism Spectrum Quotient* or AQ. This is a screening instrument in the form of a questionnaire, completed either by a parent about his or her child (e.g. the child AQ, or Adolescent AQ) or by self-report (if the adult is 'high functioning'). Examples of 10 items from the AQ (adult version) are given in Table 3.1, and the full version is available in Appendix 1.

If you answer Disagree (or Strongly Disagree) to items 1, 3, 8 and 10, that would get you 4 points on the AQ (i.e. four autistic traits). If you answer Agree (or Strongly Agree) to the other items, that would get you another 6 points on the AQ (i.e. now you are up to 10 autistic traits). There are 50 items like this in total, so everyone ends up with a score on the AQ somewhere between 0 and 50. When these are administered to a large population, the results resemble a 'normal distribution'.

A normal distribution is the bell curve that describes many traits or characteristics in which variability is seen across a population. We are familiar with this in terms of physical characteristics such as height, where most people fall in the middle of the distribution, and where one finds a

Table 3.1 Ten items from the adult version of the AQ (Autism Spectrum Quotient)

1.	I prefer to do things with others rather than on my own.
2.	I prefer to do things the same way over and over again.
3.	If I try to imagine something, I find it very easy to create a picture in my mind.
4.	I frequently get so strongly absorbed in one thing that I lose sight of other things.
5.	I often notice small sounds when others do not.
6.	I usually notice car number plates or similar strings of information.
7.	Other people frequently tell me that what I've said is impolite, even though I think it is polite.
8.	When I'm reading a story, I can easily imagine what the characters might look like.
9.	I am fascinated by dates.
10.	In a social group, I can easily keep track of several different people's conversations.

diminishing number of people in each 'tail' of the distribution (few people are very tall or very short). Equally, we are familiar with the normal distribution in terms of mental characteristics such as IQ, where again most people fall in the middle of the distribution and only a small proportion fall at the extremes. What the AQ showed, for the first time, is that autistic traits are also normally distributed across the population.

Figure 3.1 shows that at the very centre of this is the 'mean' or average for the population (designated by the symbol x). On each side of the x are vertical lines indicating 'standard deviations' (SD) from the mean. By convention we define the average range for a population as being within 1 SD above or below the mean. As Figure 3.1 shows, 34 per cent of the population fall between the mean and 1 SD above the mean, and another 34 per cent fall between the mean and 1 SD below it. So, a useful definition of 'average' or 'normality' captures 68 per cent of the population.

A more conservative definition of the average range or normality would say that anyone falling within 2 SDs of the mean is still average. As can be seen, 94 per cent of the population fall within 2 SDs of the mean (47 per cent above and 47 per cent below). Clinically, we might want to hold back and only say someone is extreme if they are outside this range (i.e. the remaining 3 per cent at each extreme).

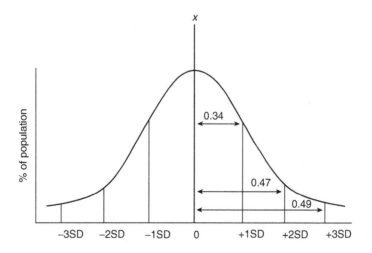

Figure 3.1 The normal (bell-shaped) distribution curve.

So, what does it mean to say that autistic traits are normally distributed in the population? As Figure 3.2 shows, it would appear that we all have some autistic traits—just like we all have some height. The AQ scale goes from zero up to a maximum of 50. As can be seen, most people without a diagnosis (the dotted line) fall in the range 0–25. Since the mean for the general population is 16.0 and 1 SD is 3 points, then taking the definition of average as falling within 2 SDs from the mean would lead us to the conclusion that scores between 10 and 23 are 'average'.

What Figure 3.2 also shows is that most people with a diagnosis of an autism spectrum condition (the continuous line) fall in the range of 26–50. Eighty per cent of them score above 32, and 99 per cent score above 26. So the AQ neatly separates the groups: 93 per cent of the general population fall in the average range of the AQ, and 99 per cent of the autistic population fall in the extreme (high end) of the scale.

Notice, however, that there is some overlap. What this means is that there are some people *without* a diagnosis who score in the extreme range, and some people with a diagnosis who fall in the average range. This reminds us that the AQ is not diagnostic—it is a screening instrument—and that a diagnosis is only given if a person is *suffering* to some degree. Having an autism spectrum condition remains a medical diagnosis that should not be trivialized. So, one could have two individuals who both have an AQ score at the same point

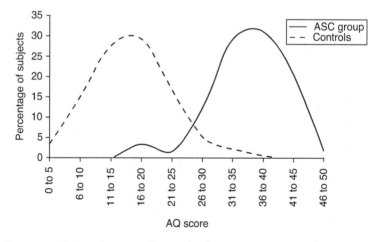

Figure 3.2 AQ scores in a group diagnosed with Autism Spectrum Conditions (ASC), and a typical control group.

(say, both scoring 35 out of 50); yet one might need a diagnosis whilst the other might not. This is likely to reflect a range of factors, such as the degree of support the person is receiving, or the additional presence of learning difficulties, or language difficulties.

A closer look at the AQ reveals some subtle individual differences. For example, in Figure 3.3, we can see that in the general population, males score slightly (but significantly) higher than females. It is only a 2 point difference (females have an average AQ score of 15 and males of 17), but it may be telling us something important. Autism spectrum conditions are far more common in males than in females (classic autism occurs in four males for every one female, and Asperger syndrome occurs in nine males for every one female). The finding that (in a general population) males naturally have more autistic traits than females suggests that the number of autistic traits a person has is linked to a sex-linked biological factor (genetic or hormonal, or both). This is a point we will return to in Chapter 6, when we consider the biological causes of autism and Asperger syndrome.

So far we have seen that people with an autism spectrum condition score very high on the AQ, and that there are sex differences on the AQ in the general population. This scale also allows us to look for other groups who score differently in terms of number of autistic traits. One such group are the first-degree relatives (such as siblings or parents) of children with an autism spectrum

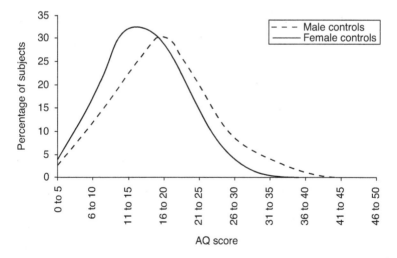

Figure 3.3 Sex differences on the AQ in the general population.

Table 3.2 Average AQ scores of different groups in the population. (The range is 3 points above or below each average.)

AQ score	Group
32+	Autism spectrum condition
26	First-degree relatives with the 'broader autism phenotype'[1]
17	Males
15	Females

condition, who score mid-way between those with the condition and those without. This is shown in Table 3.2.

This indicates that whilst the AQ is a continuous distribution, different factors (related to your biological sex, or your genetic relationship to someone with autism or Asperger syndrome) can increase your AQ score. The new conceptualization of the autistic spectrum as continuous throughout the general population is shown in Figure 3.4.

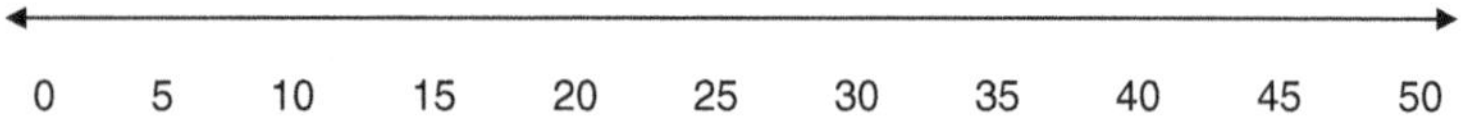

| 0 | 5 | 10 | 15 | 20 | 25 | 30 | 35 | 40 | 45 | 50 |

Figure 3.4 The new conceptualization: autistic traits run right through the population. (The scale shows AQ points with no categorical diagnoses.)

Why do so many more males receive a diagnosis of autism or Asperger syndrome?

Harvard psychologist Steven Pinker reminds us that there is a surprising mathematical property of the normal distribution. If two groups (e.g. males and females) differ a bit at the centre of the range (in their means), then because the rate at which the slope of the curve falls off, at the extremes the differences between the groups will be huge! So, for example, with height, the two sexes differ by 3 inches on average. At 5 feet 10 inches, the sex ratio is 30:1 (male:female). In people just 2 inches taller (6 feet), the sex ratio jumps up to a 2000:1!

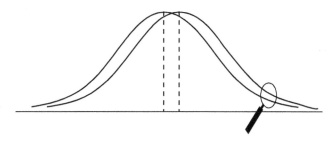

Figure 3.5 Two groups (e.g. males and females) differ in their average scores.

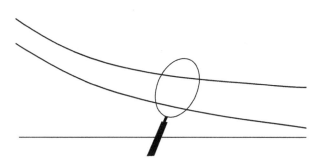

Figure 3.6 At the extremes, the two groups (e.g. males and females) differ much more. (This is because the curve falls off as a negative exponential of the square of the distance from the mean).

In Figure 3.6, we can see quite why this is happening, thanks to the magnifying glass (shown in the right-hand tail of Figure 3.5 with the area enlarged in Figure 3.6). What now becomes apparent is that the gap between the sexes widens as we move to the extremes. And because this is a purely statistical property (i.e., the statistical rules apply whether we are talking about any continuous dimension that is normally distributed), this will apply as much to height or blood pressure as to autistic traits.

Such detailed analysis of scores on measures of autistic traits reveal the *dimensional* nature of autism, but the diagnosis of autism and Asperger Syndrome remains categorical. We turn to look at this next.

4

Making the diagnosis

➲ Key points

- The diagnosis of autism and Asperger syndrome is often carried out by a multidisciplinary team, typically taking 2 or 3 hours, based on interview and observation. Classic autism is thankfully usually diagnosed by the age of 3, and can be diagnosed as young as 18 months. Asperger syndrome is often not diagnosed until at least 6, and often much later than this, including late diagnosis in adulthood.

- In the future, biological markers may enable diagnosis to be more objective. When any claims emerge for a biologically based diagnostic test, there will need to be research to establish if the test has good specificity (does the test just identify people with autism spectrum conditions, or does it also identify people with other conditions?) and good sensitivity (how many cases does the test identify correctly, how many does it miss, and how many does it identify incorrectly?).

- Diagnosis is only of value when it is not just a label but a passport into accessing all the necessary support services that each individual may need.

We have covered some of the history of autism and Asperger syndrome, and been introduced to the concept of autistic traits lying on a continuum. But for some readers of this book, the urgent question in their mind is where to obtain a diagnosis and what to expect from the doctor making the diagnosis. Appendix 2 contains a list of all the autism and Asperger syndrome associations that we know about throughout the world, who could direct you to a clinic local to you. Irrespective of whether you are the parent of a young child with suspected autism or Asperger syndrome, or are an adult with suspected Asperger syndrome, the diagnostic assessment has a typical format that involves asking questions to collect information around three key questions:

1. Does the person have significant *social* difficulties?

The clinician conducting the diagnostic interview (who might be a child psychiatrist, clinical or educational psychologist, paediatrician or other health professional) might ask you questions such as (but not restricted to) the following:

- Have they found it difficult to make and keep friends?

- Have they found it hard to understand and respond appropriately to other people's feelings?

- Can they join in larger, unstructured social groups (not just one-to-one social interaction)?

- Are they socially withdrawn?

- Do they tend to misinterpret other's intentions?

- Do they use *eye contact* inappropriately, either staring at others for too long, or looking at other people's eyes too briefly, or at the wrong times?

- Do they show a lack of normal *social awareness*?

- Are they to some extent oblivious of what others are thinking about them, or how they come across to others?

- Would they spontaneously comfort another person?

- Can they pick up on other people's feelings, not just using the extreme cues (such as someone crying), but using more subtle cues (e.g. to determine if someone is pretending to be happy)?

- In the second year of life, was there a delay in showing *joint attention* (such as following where others are looking, or using the pointing gesture to share interest or following another person pointing to share interest)?

- Have they always been more comfortable in solitary pursuits?

These latter two examples are to determine if social difficulties have been present right across the person's development, from infancy onwards.

2. The person's *communication* skills.

As mentioned in Chapter 1, social and communication skills cannot be truly separated, but for the diagnosis the clinician may try to cover these separately. The kinds of interviewing questions that they might ask include (but are not restricted to) the following:

- Does the person have a very *literal* understanding of language?
- Does the person have trouble understanding non-literal language (such as humour, sarcasm, irony and metaphor)?
- Is there a noticeable difference between the person's technical language skills (e.g. their vocabulary, or their syntactic ability) and their *pragmatic* language skills (i.e. being able to use language appropriately to the social context)?
- Does the person frequently say (as well as do) the wrong thing in a social situation (committing *faux pas*)?
- Do they tend to provide either *too little* information or *too much* information in their speech (or e-mails or other written communication)? Being able to judge what the listener needs to know is part of being able to take the other person's perspective into account.
- Do they have trouble with *turn-taking* in language, tending to hold forth in a monologue (and not realize that others are getting bored)?
- Was there any *delay* in their language skills? (Recall from Chapter 1 that a sign of delay is relevant to distinguishing classic autism from Asperger syndrome.) Delay is typically defined when the child is not using single words by 2 years old, or any phrase speech by 3 years old.
- Was the pattern of language acquisition atypical? For example, were first words highly unusual, such as being unusually specific or rare words?

3. The person's narrow, unusual and strong interests, as well as unusually repetitive behaviour.

The clinician might ask questions such as (but not confined to) the following:

- Has the person—right across their life—been capable of becoming *totally immersed* in one activity or interest to the exclusion of all else, concentrating for many hours each day on just one unusual topic?
- Did they tend to become an expert on that topic?

(continued)

- Would that topic have the quality of an *obsession*, in that efforts by others to shift the person on to new activities failed?

- Have they had a strong need to do the same thing over and over again, in a highly similar way? For example, positioning objects in the house and becoming very upset if other people moved them? Or taking the same route to school or work? Or performing some activity in a strict sequence that they refuse to change?

- Would they have become very upset if they had had to deviate from this routine?

- Do they invariably go through the *same* sequence of actions when beginning certain activities?

- Do they insist on wearing the *same* clothes, or eating the same food or going to the same places, over and over again?

- Do they resist change?

These latter characteristics, for me, go to the heart of autism and Asperger syndrome. Kanner identified this as the person's *need for sameness.* At other times he referred to it as their *resistance to change.* It is almost as if, just as a Type 1 diabetic starts to suffer if their blood sugar level rises too quickly, a person with autism or Asperger syndrome starts to suffer if they encounter unexpected change. We will see in Chapter 5 how this 'symptom' has been explained in terms of the person's strong drive to *systemize* events, to render them as near to predictable as they can. Anything that occurs in an unpredictable way is likely to throw the person into a panic and may trigger a withdrawal or an avoidance, or a desperate attempt to re-establish predictability by imposing a fixed pattern or sequence of behaviour.

The structured interview is conducted with a view to establishing if the person's behaviour in each of these three areas is significantly unusual, and if their difficulties in each of the three areas have interfered with everyday functioning. The interview is usually complemented by direct observation, in order to gather direct evidence in each of these areas of atypical behaviour.

Standardized instruments

When diagnosing a child, it is increasingly usual to use a standardized method such as the ADI (*Autism Diagnostic Interview*) and/or the ADOS (the *Autism Diagnostic Observational Schedule*). These methods were developed by Michael Rutter in London and Cathy Lord in Michigan, and are sometimes referred to as the 'gold standard' in diagnosis. Clinicians have to pay to be trained in these methods, and training takes about 1 week. During this training and after it, the trainee is assessed for how accurately they have learnt to make the diagnosis, i.e. how reliably they agree with other trained clinicians.

Such standardization of diagnostic methods was important to attempt, because previously all that was available was 'clinical judgement' or the doctor's opinion. However, the latest research shows that these methods are not a gold standard in that they work best when combined with 'clinical opinion'. That is, the original hope that they could replace the subjective opinion of the doctor has not turned out to be the case, because they miss some cases of Asperger syndrome. They are also less useful for the assessment of adults, though there are some standardized methods available for this purpose, such as the *Adult Asperger Assessment* (AAA). The *Diagnostic Instrument for Social and Communication Disorders* (DISCO) is another useful alternative, developed by Dr Lorna Wing.

One day, the hope is that accurate diagnosis will not depend on the vagaries of a clinical interview or of direct observation of behaviour, which invariably includes some subjective elements. Instead, it will be based on a biological marker or set of markers (e.g. a combination of specific gene variants, or a combination of specific protein levels), measured in the blood or in other bodily tissue or cells. But for now, such a set of biological markers for autism or Asperger syndrome is not yet available, so we need to continue to rely on behavioural and interview-based methods.

Intelligence tests (IQ), and related educational and cognitive measures

It is important that the clinic has some measure of the person's overall IQ, since for the diagnosis of Asperger syndrome the person must have an IQ in the average (or above average) range, i.e. have no signs of general learning difficulties. We discussed in Chapter 2 how different IQ bands in some sense enable a clinician to refine the subgroup into which the person's diagnosis falls. IQ is also important because it remains a very strong predictor of prognosis, and because the specific profile on an IQ test (e.g. strengths in visual spatial tests or difficulties in verbal tests) can be used to plan individual educational programmes for the child.

For a child, it is also important to have a measure of language ability (both comprehension and expression): recall that the diagnosis of Asperger syndrome is only made if the person shows no signs of language delay. Noting the size of the language delay will also be of practical importance in planning interventions such as speech therapy for a child with classic autism. Finally, in some clinics, the doctor will undertake some other psychological tests (of everyday planning abilities, or of memory, for example) not because these are intrinsic to the diagnosis (they are not) but because they might help to understand the person's unique pattern of strengths and difficulties.

What to expect when you go for a diagnostic assessment

Most clinics use a multidisciplinary team. What this means is that you might expect a mix of professionals in the interview or in the room observing you or your child. As mentioned earlier, these might include a child psychiatrist, clinical psychologist, speech therapist, educational psychologist, paediatrician or other related disciplines (neurologists, for example). Sometimes in order not to be too overwhelming, the team may observe behind a one-way mirror, always with your prior knowledge and consent.

Typically a diagnostic assessment takes at least 2–3 hours, and in some clinics it takes a whole day, with breaks. The team should be able to give you the outcome (a diagnosis if appropriate) on the same day, and you should try to prepare some questions to ask the team, in the event that they confirm the diagnosis is on the autistic spectrum. That way, you make the most of being with the specialists, and can benefit the most from their advice.

What should happen immediately following a diagnosis

People react differently to hearing the words 'I think your child has autism' or 'I think you have Asperger syndrome'. Some are relieved that finally there is a name for the condition that has always made them feel they, or their child, are different; and relieved that finally they have a signpost for where to go for the most relevant help. Some react with a sense of shock that they, or their child, have a condition that is understood to be genetic, affecting brain development (see Chapter 6). The shock can sometimes turn to sadness if hopes turn to disappointments about the future. People vary in how quickly they adjust to the diagnosis.

The clinician giving you the diagnosis should tell you about the National Autistic Society (NAS) in the UK, the Autism Society of America (ASA) in the US, or the equivalent in your state or country (see Appendix 2 for a list of such associations). These associations mostly began as parent-led charities and in many countries have become powerful lobbying groups, running services such as special schools, adult day centres, sheltered housing or sheltered employment services, social groups, playgroups, etc.

For many people with an autism spectrum condition, it is possible to see the diagnosis in a positive light. It is a statement that the person has followed an atypical path of brain development. In the language of people with Asperger syndrome, they are not 'neurotypical'. As we will see in Chapter 5, the psychology of autism and Asperger syndrome involves areas of strength as well as areas of difficulties. The difficulties (in socializing and communicating through small-talk) can be disabling unless environments are chosen to minimize this. But the strengths (in attention to detail, the ability to concentrate for hours and hours on a single topic, the thoroughness with which narrow topics are explored and the systematic approach to certain activities) can be great assets if they can be harnessed usefully (in education, in work, or in hobbies, for example).

Where to find help and support

The list of agencies at the end of this book may provide a useful starting point for support groups near you.

How early can a diagnosis be made?

Autism can be reliably diagnosed by 18 months of age. Many clinics are unaware that this is possible, but studies have been conducted showing that diagnoses made at that age using the established instruments such as the ADI and ADOS are reliable, and predict later diagnosis.

Some Health Visitors and GPs/paediatricians use screening instruments such as the Checklist for Autism in Toddlers (CHAT), which look for the absence of behaviours that one would expect to be present in a typically developing toddler (such as joint attention) as well as the presence of behaviours that are not usually present in a typically developing toddler (such as rocking back and forth for hours). The CHAT has been modified into the Modified-CHAT (M-CHAT) and the Quantitative-CHAT (Q-CHAT). [See http://www.utismresearchcentre.com for the latter.] These are not diagnostic, but help to indicate if a child might warrant a full diagnostic assessment.

Will my child grow out of it? What will happen to him or her when they grow up?

Autism and Asperger syndrome are life-long in that they reflect the make up of the brain. Whilst the brain changes and adapts, ultimately the core of autism and Asperger syndrome is part of who that person is. In the case of Asperger syndrome we can think of the condition as being a form of personality type. It is possible to adapt your personality to the outside world when needed, but one's personality ultimately is who you are, and aspects of the core (such as excellent attention to detail or sensory hyper-sensitivity) do not fundamentally change across one's life. For some people, social skills improve to varying degrees, with age and experience.

Can the diagnosis be removed later?

A person who receives a diagnosis will not necessarily need that diagnosis all their lives. A diagnosis is made at a particular snapshot in time, at a point in that person's life when things had got so difficult that they needed the diagnosis in order to access support and help.

In the case of Asperger syndrome it may, for example, have been useful to have a diagnosis as a teenager, when they weren't coping with mainstream school and the social pressures that this implies. By adulthood, that same person might have found a niche in which they not only feel they fit, but in which they are thriving, and feel they no longer need the diagnosis. I have come across people who seek the diagnosis and I have come across people who seek to be undiagnosed. The latter are just as valid as the former, but will need just as thorough a reassessment of the individual. This is to check it is the case that they are coping sufficiently such that the autistic traits that they have no longer interfere with their daily life. If this is the case, then they no longer meet the criteria for a diagnosis. The clinician needs to discuss with them the pros and cons of removing the diagnosis.

In the case of classic autism, we need to be realistic that the person may need the diagnosis all of their lives. We discussed in Chapter 2 how in some sense this is the more 'severe' subgroup on the autistic spectrum. The rare exceptions to this are individuals with high-functioning autism, who in terms of daily living skills may achieve the same level of independence as someone with Asperger syndrome. But the medium- and low-functioning individuals on the autistic spectrum will need their diagnosis all their lives, to ensure they obtain help with sheltered living, sheltered employment and protection as a vulnerable person.

Horror stories

There are examples of bad practice out there, and there is still a lot of ignorance or misunderstanding about autism and Asperger syndrome. I wish this book could contain all positive stories, but to do this would be pure spin. We need to look at what is actually happening on the ground, not how things should be in an ideal world. Here are two examples that make me very worried:

* Social workers who refuse to believe that a child has autism or Asperger syndrome, and instead think the child's difficult behaviour (their social difficulties, their tantrums at change, their lack of social conformity, their learning difficulties) are signs of *inadequate parenting and neglect*, rather than signs of a neurological condition.

* Parents who are accused of *Munchausen by proxy*, a clinician's term for suggesting the parent wants his or her child to have problems, in order to satisfy some disturbed need for the attention of doctors.

I have heard of parents whose child is put on the 'at risk' register because the social workers believe such things. Such attitudes are horrific and set the clock back by 50 years in perceiving autism and Asperger syndrome as reactions to poor parenting, instead of recognizing that autism and Asperger syndrome are neurological conditions in need of sensitive support. Recall in Chapter 2 how we discussed Bettelheim's inaccurate theory (in the 1960s) about parents causing their child's autism, and Rutter's refutation of this idea (in the 1970s).

Naturally, social workers and others need to be open to the possibility of abuse or neglect, but this should not be at the cost of dismissing an alternative diagnosis. The horror cases I have come across tend to involve a dogmatic bigotry on the part of social services who may say that they do not believe that Asperger syndrome exists, or believe that there is some fashion involving over-diagnosis of Asperger syndrome, and a refusal to acknowledge such cases as genuine. The despair of such parents on the receiving end of such dismissive attitudes is heart-breaking.

I have also heard of other horror stories:

* Parents of children with autism not receiving appropriate support and feeling so desperate with a child who does not sleep, cannot adjust to change, and is occasionally even aggressive, that the parent attempts suicide or actually commits suicide. Such tragedies are preventable with a little bit of humanity and care on the part of local services.

◆ Adults with Asperger syndrome who, having got the diagnosis, find that their local services do nothing. Such adults sometimes decide that since no-one cares, and they have slipped into a depression, they will end their own life. Again, such suicides are preventable if agencies are properly 'joined up'.

◆ The local services sometimes pass the buck by saying that Asperger syndrome is the responsibility of the local mental health team. They in turn say that Asperger syndrome is not a mental health condition but a learning disability. The learning disabilities team then say that Asperger syndrome is not a learning disability because the person has an IQ above 70 and is an educational responsibility. The educational authority may then pass the buck by saying it is a social services responsibility, who pass the responsibility back to the mental health team. You can see how this can go round and round in circles, whilst the person with Asperger syndrome feels more and more isolated.

Parents still need to be advocates for their child with autism

From the above, it will become apparent that our world is still not as autism- or Asperger-friendly as it could be. Until it is, parents and others continue to have a role in educating their local school, social services, GP or education authority about the nature of autism and Asperger syndrome, and in fighting on behalf of their child for appropriate support. They should not have to take on this role, because they may already have a lot of stress to deal with. Realistically, it is important to recognize that such parental involvement may be essential in helping a person with autism or Asperger syndrome get the right support. Joining a parent support group can make it feel less like having to fight alone.

Students with Asperger syndrome

There are other equally avoidable sad outcomes, such as students with Asperger syndrome dropping out of university because the university system is not being flexible in making allowances for their Asperger syndrome. I know for example of students with Asperger syndrome whose learning style is more suited to private study (from textbooks, or from journal articles available via electronic libraries on the web), but who are required to attend lectures and seminars as part of their degree.

Lectures and seminars were not designed for people with Asperger syndrome, because these educational formats typically

- involve large social groups

- are noisy

- expect the student to edit what the lecturer is saying into short-hand notes

- expect the student to switch topics after 55 minutes

- expect the student to do two things (listening and writing) at once

- expect the student to sit in any available place

- expect the student to concentrate even with whispering from other students.

In contrast, many students with Asperger syndrome may

- prefer to work in silence

- prefer to go slowly and methodically

- prefer not to have to edit (for fear of losing important detail)

- prefer to error-check, to be sure that a fact is a fact

- prefer conditions to remain unchanged (same seat, same lighting, etc.)

- prefer lack of distractions

- prefer to see all of the logical steps or evidence for each statement, rather than accepting assertions in the absence of explanations

- prefer, once they start a topic, to stay on that topic for many hours, ignoring lunch or drinks or even the need to go to the bathroom

- become irritated by the intrusion of other people into their space

- become anxious if other people talk to them unexpectedly

- become irritated by human errors in lecture handouts

- become irritated by a chatty style of lecturing

- become irritated by the whispering students in the row behind them in the lecture theatre who want to talk about who is going out with whom.

Universities are places of learning, and there should not be a dogmatic attitude that assumes that all students learn in the same way. Some students will learn best through lectures, but others will learn best far away from the hustle and bustle of lecture theatres or even seminar groups.

The authorities need to keep in mind that many people with Asperger syndrome dream of a planet where they are the only human being, where there are no interruptions, where events happen with regularity and predictability. Many pine for the lifestyles that were adopted by monks in monasteries, where a calm tranquility allowed for routines in domestic life combined with solitary work. If universities want students with Asperger syndrome to come to study, they need to accept that all that matters is that the person is learning.

How they learn should not be the purview of the university governing body. *What* they are examined in is a reasonable area for universities to legislate on, and the test of the student will still be in exam performance, alongside all other students. The student with Asperger syndrome may require a quiet room away from the hundreds of other students in which to take his or her exam papers. Thankfully, many universities now have a Disability Resource Centre with specialists in Asperger syndrome, who can help assess what such students need in order to ensure that they enjoy their years in college and fulfil their potential.

Prenatal screening and diagnosis: potential benefits and dangers

Let us return to the main focus of this chapter: diagnosis. What will have become apparent is that diagnosis is still based on behavioural criteria. This is true for most of psychiatry, where we still do not have diagnostic biological markers for most conditions. (The exceptions to this are some of the learning disabilities, such as Down syndrome, and some of the dementias.)

There are some questions about how biological markers, if they were available to detect autism or Asperger syndrome, would be used or abused. In the final section of this chapter, we explore some of the ethical issues this raises. If it were possible to diagnose purely on the basis of genes or proteins, for example, this could open the door to *prenatal* diagnosis, or at least prenatal *screening*. Just as it is now possible to screen for Down syndrome using the 'triple test' (a blood test from the pregnant mother) or to detect Down syndrome using *amniocentesis* during pregnancy (during which some of the amniotic fluid in which the foetus is bathed is sampled using a long needle, because this fluid contains lots of cells from the foetus itself), so it might one day be possible to screen or detect autism or Asperger syndrome from a maternal blood test or foetal amniotic fluid test.

Currently the results of such tests for Down syndrome are used to enable parents to make a decision about whether to continue with the pregnancy or opt for a termination. The fear from at least some of the higher-functioning individuals with autism or with Asperger syndrome is that these methods, if and when they become available, could lead to *prevention* of autism or Asperger syndrome, or to some form of *eugenics* (genetic and social engineering). Understandably, those who feel autism or Asperger syndrome is a central part of their identity, or who feel it is responsible for their strengths (not just their difficulties), feel this is a major threat to their very existence, and that society would lose potentially valuable genes from the gene pool.

We will see in Chapters 5 and 6 how the genes for autism and Asperger syndrome not only lead to difficulties but (in some of the other family members, or even in those with a diagnosis) may lead to talents in areas such as exceptional attention to detail, ability to focus deeply to develop expertise, extraordinary memory and remarkable ability to detect patterns (useful in fields such as maths, music, engineering, craftsmanship and the 'hard' sciences). In this way, the fears expressed by some people with Asperger syndrome are not just about their civil liberties—their right to life—but also about the relationship between the genes underlying autism and Asperger syndrome, and the genes that have enabled human beings to produce great art, science and technology.

On the other side of the argument are parents' right to choose whether to continue with a pregnancy or not, especially if the child is likely to have major disabilities such as severe learning difficulties. A second argument in support of prenatal screening is the potential for such methods to enable early intervention to be provided, in theory from birth. That is, prenatal screening does not have to lead to termination; it can lead to early intervention.

The latter argument is, for me, one of the most important reasons for pushing ahead with research into prenatal diagnosis, since at present many children (and adults) have to wait far too long to obtain their diagnosis. If the means were available, it could then be determined if early intervention (beginning in infancy) leads to a greater reduction in later difficulties, compared with intervention that begins later. We return to the whole topic of intervention in Chapter 7.

The other major benefit of research into prenatal factors (e.g., as genes, or hormones produced by the foetus) is to help us understand the fundamental causes of autism and Asperger syndrome. Greater understanding of causal factors is important in any area of science and medicine. The above discussion is necessary to flag up the ethical issues surrounding this area, so that there is proper debate and caution in how science and clinical practice proceed.

5

The psychology of autism and Asperger syndrome

Key points

The five major psychological theories of autism and Asperger syndrome are:

- Executive dysfunction theory

- Weak central coherence theory

- Mindblindness theory

- Empathizing–systemizing theory [and by extension, the extreme male brain theory]

- Magnocellular theory

Psychological theories need to explain all autistic traits in all individuals on the spectrum, not just some of them. They ultimately also need to integrate with neurobiological theories.

Five major theories have been put forward to understand the behaviour and psychological profile of people with autism and Asperger syndrome. In this chapter, we consider the evidence for each theory, before undertaking a comparison of how well each of the five theories accounts for the whole range of autistic traits.

The executive dysfunction theory

Executive function is defined as the ability to control action. Actions may be 'motor', (i.e., movements), attention and even thoughts. Action control includes creating plans, executing plans, staying on topic and shifting attention as required. According to this first theory, the core features of people on the autistic spectrum are best explained by an inability to plan actions (executive control) and shift attention.

Executive dysfunction is characteristic of patients who have suffered damage to the prefrontal cortex. The idea is that, whilst in autism there has been no obvious damage to the frontal lobes, *developmentally* the prefrontal cortex may not have matured in the typical way.

According to this theory, this can explain the repetitive behaviour in autism, since if you cannot plan actions or shift attention, your behaviour would become 'stuck' in the same groove, unable to move flexibly onto a new plan or path. You would, according to this theory, be destined to repeat or *perseverate*.

The evidence for this theory is limited. There are some reports of people with autism who take longer on the Tower of London Test (see Figure 5.1),

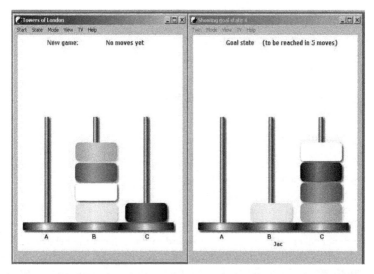

Figure 5.1 The Tower of London Test of executive dysfunction. Move the discs from the starting configuration to the goal configuration in as few moves as possible. (This can be done in 5 moves at a minimum).

where you have to move the discs from the starting pattern to the target pattern in the fewest number of moves. However, there are other reports of people with Asperger syndrome who can perform very well on this test. This suggests it cannot explain everyone on the autistic spectrum. In addition, there are many clinical groups who perform badly on this test, so difficulties on it are not specific to the autistic spectrum.

The executive dysfunction theory has also been tested using tests of verbal fluency, for example asking the person to name as many words beginning with a target letter (e.g. S) as one can in 1 minute. People with autism or Asperger syndrome are less good at generating such lists, though this may be because they organize their memories in a more interesting way than in alphabetical lists.

A further criticism of this theory is that the narrow interests or 'obsessions' are presumed to reflect some inability to shift attention to new topics, leading to some dysfunctional tendency to get stuck. As such, this theory ignores the *content* of the narrow interests, seeing the obsessions as random. In contrast, the hyper-systemizing theory (described below) sees the narrow interests not as the result of some pathology but as the result of a remarkable depth of processing, a tendency to go deeper into the details of a topic, compared with the typical brain. It also sees the content of such narrow interests as non-random, but specifically drawn to information that is systemizable. The result is the development of areas of expertise.

Nevertheless, the executive dysfunction theory has some strengths. It captures well the difficulty that some people with autism have in shifting attention. The term executive dysfunction may need revising so as to specify that people with autism or Asperger syndrome are remarkably good at *inhibiting* all other stimuli outside their narrow spotlight of attention.

Personally, I would like to see the executive dysfunction theory connect with a related theory called the *Monotropism* theory. According to monotropism, the typical brain can multitask and keep a dual focus in mind simultaneously. The person with autism or Asperger syndrome may be less able to multitask, leaving their attention with a single focus. This needs to be fully tested, but I think it has a lot of truth to it.

Weak central coherence

According to this second theory, people on the autistic spectrum have problems in integrating information to make a coherent, global picture. Instead, they are said to focus on the small, local details in a scene. Thus, whereas the neurotypical mind has strong central coherence, more likely to attend to the gist rather than the nitty-gritty, the autistic mind is said to have weak central coherence, more likely to attend to the detail than to the overview.

This theory is attractive because it offers an explanation for the *islets of ability* in autism and Asperger syndrome: the excellent attention to detail, memory for detail, and skills in a narrow topic. The evidence for weak central coherence is stronger than the evidence for the executive dysfunction theory. First, people on the autistic spectrum are faster on the Children's (Figure 5.2) or the Adult Embedded Figures Test (Figure 5.3). On these tests, you are asked to find the target shape as quickly as you can, hidden in the larger design.

Also, on the Navon Test (Figure 5.4), people with autism spectrum conditions are more likely to report that they see the letter H rather than the letter A, suggesting they have a preference to perceive the local rather than the global image.

A final example of a test of this theory is the homographs tests, in which the person being tested is asked to read sentences that contain a homograph (a word that has two possible pronunciations, the correct one depending on the sentence context). An example is 'She had a *tear* in her eye' and 'She had a *tear* in her dress'. According to at least one study, people with autism or Asperger syndrome are more likely to mispronounce the key word *tear*. Presumably this is because they are overfocused on each individual word in the sentence, but not simultaneously attending to the wider context (the meaning of the whole sentence) in which this word occurs.

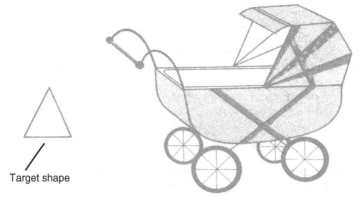

Target shape

Figure 5.2 The Children's Embedded Figures Test: where is the same triangle?

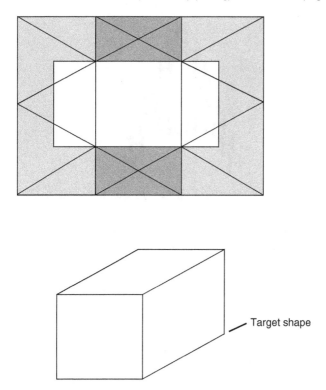

Target shape

Figure 5.3 The Adult Embedded Figures Test: where is the same cube?

I like this theory because it draws to our notice the fact that people with autism spectrum conditions have superior attention for smaller details compared with people without autism spectrum conditions. It also reminds us that people with autism or Asperger syndrome may take longer to make use of the wider context, the bigger picture, instead focusing on smaller units of information.

One shortcoming of this theory, however, is that it implies that people with autism or Asperger syndrome cannot see the whole, which cannot be true. If you ask them if they can see the big letter A in the Navon test (see Figure 5.4),

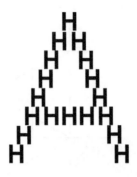

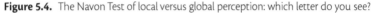

Figure 5.4. The Navon Test of local versus global perception: which letter do you see?

they can of course see it perfectly well. This theory, to be successful, will have to clarify at exactly which level this difficulty with integration of information is meant to occur. Clearly it doesn't occur at the basic level of featural integration or the letter T would not be seen as an T but instead as a I and a ⌐. Nor is there what is called a 'binding' problem, preventing them from seeing objects as objects rather than as clusters of features. I suspect that the difficulties with integration occur at a higher level.

One way in which the weak central coherence theory could be revised is to link itself with a neurological theory that we will encounter in the next chapter, called the *connectivity* theory. This states that in autism and Asperger syndrome there is short-range overconnectivity (more nerve cells or neurons making lots of local connections in the brain) but long-range underconnectivity (fewer neurons making connections between more distant brain areas).

A second way in which weak central coherence could be taken forward is to link with the growing evidence for *sensory hypersensitivity* in autism and Asperger syndrome. There are plenty of clinical anecdotes of people with autism and Asperger syndrome reacting to small differences between objects, or noticing details that others do not. There is also experimental evidence that children and adults with ASC are faster and more accurate on *visual search tasks*. Several studies suggest that people on the autistic spectrum are quicker to detect changes in sound, touch and vision, and that this may extend to smell too. This might reflect a very basic difference at the level of neurophysiology in autism and Asperger syndrome, which has not yet been isolated. This is sometimes referred to as 'enhanced perceptual function'.

The sensory hypersensitivity theory clearly has major implications for creating autism- and Asperger-friendly environments (at school, at home or at work), to minimize the stress from unpleasant sensory distractions (such as neon lights flickering, clocks ticking, and radios playing even at a distance).

The mindblindness theory

This third theory proposes that children with autism spectrum conditions are delayed in developing a *theory of mind*. A theory of mind (ToM) is the ability to put oneself into someone else's shoes, to imagine their thoughts and feelings, so as to be able to make sense of and predict their behaviour. It is sometimes also called *mind-reading* or *mentalizing*.

So, when we see someone else turn to look out of the window, we typically infer that they must have *seen* something of *interest*, and that they might *know* about something that we cannot presently see. It might even be something that they *want*. Notice that in this interpretation, we have gone beyond mere behaviour to imagine a whole set of *mental states* that link up in the other person's mind. When we mindread or use a ToM, we can not only make sense of another person's behaviour (why did their head swivel on their neck? Why did their eyes move left?), but we can predict what they might do next. (If they want what they just saw, they are likely to move towards it. If they fear what they just saw, they are likely to move away from it.)

It is in this sense that ToM can be thought of as a theory: it explains and predicts others' behaviour. People with autism or Asperger syndrome may be puzzled by other people's actions, or anxious because other people's behaviour seems unpredictable, precisely because they cannot use a ToM to interpret or anticipate what others are doing or are going to do.

We also use our ToM to identify people's *intentions* behind their gestures and their speech. So, for example, when we see one person look at another and then look at the door, we can infer that one person may be communicating to another that it is time to leave. They want their audience to recognize their intention that in moving their eyes in a particular direction, this means 'Let's go!' Or if a person says 'We'll cross that bridge when we get to it', they intend their listener to understand that this means 'Let's not worry about that until it happens'. People with autism or Asperger syndrome may wonder why one person is looking at another in a certain way, or may take language literally, conjuring up pictures of bridges in their mind when they hear an expression like the one above. In doing so, they reveal that they are not picking up on the other person's intentions—they are not using their ToM.

This theory proposes that children with autism and Asperger syndrome are delayed in the development of their ToM, leaving them with degrees of *mindblindness*. As a consequence, they find other people's behaviour confusing and unpredictable, even frightening. Evidence for this comes from difficulties they show at each point in the development of the capacity to mindread. Here are the key stages in typical development:

- A typical 14-month-old child shows *joint attention* (such as pointing or following another person's gaze), during which they not only look at another person's face and eyes, but pay attention to what the other person is interested in. Children with autism and Asperger syndrome show reduced frequency of joint attention, in toddlerhood. They point less, look up at faces less and do not turn to follow another person's gaze as much as a typical child.

- The typical 24-month-old child can engage in *pretend play*. When they interact with someone else who is pretending, they need to use their mind-reading skills to be able to understand that in the other person's mind, they are just pretending. Children with autism and Asperger syndrome show less pretend play, or their pretence is limited to more rule-based formats. For example, they may simply follow a make-believe script from a movie, or science fiction, where the pretend world is specified in terms of a set of 'facts' about that pretend universe.

- The typical 3-year-old child can pass the *seeing leads to knowing* test, depicted in Figure 5.5. To pass the test question, the child needs to notice that whilst Sally touched the box, Anne actually *looked* into it, and since seeing is one way to get knowledge, Anne is the one who must know what's in the box. Children with autism and Asperger syndrome are delayed in passing this test.

This principle of *seeing leads to knowing* is part of the intuitive understanding typical children have about how other people's minds work. They are not formally taught such principles, but pick them up by interacting in a social environment, probably because their brain is programmed to develop such knowledge rapidly. Children with autism spectrum conditions often need to be taught such principles explicitly, because they are not picking them up naturally. (A useful resource for teachers in this area is called *Teaching Children with Autism to Mind-read: A Practical Guide*, published by Wiley in 1999.)

- The typical 4-year-old child can pass the 'false belief' test, depicted in Figure 5.6. On this test, you have to follow a short story about two dolls (again called Sally and Anne). The child being tested is told that 'Sally hides her marble in the box, but when Sally goes out, naughty Anne moves the marble to the basket'. At the end of this short story, the child is asked 'Where will Sally look for her marble?'

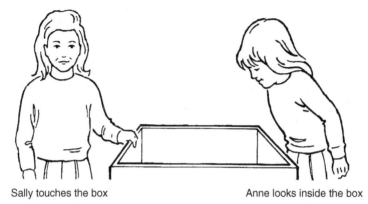

Sally touches the box   Anne looks inside the box

Figure 5.5 The Seeing Leads to Knowing Test: which one knows what's in the box?

The typical 4-year-old says that Sally will look for it where she left it, i.e. in the box, since this is Sally's *false belief* about the location of the marble. In contrast, most children with autism and Asperger syndrome say that Sally will look where the marble actually is, i.e. in the basket, even though there is no way she could know that it had moved. In this sense, they fail to demonstrate that they can take another person's point of view.

A more everyday example of being able to use a ToM (or engage in mind-reading) comes from the children's story *Snow White*, where even the typical 4-year-old child can understand that Snow White is being deceived by her wicked godmother who wants her to *believe* the apple is tasty, whilst all the while it contains poison.

A lot of children's and even adult's drama hinges on what one person knows or doesn't know, as a way of creating an interesting plot, with suspense. Many such plots can be wasted on children with autism spectrum conditions, who may be excellent at tracking the physical details and changes in a scene or a story, but fail to read the implicit level of characters' motivational, emotional and informational states of mind. The Snow White example also reminds us that mindreading is not only important when it comes to making sense of and predicting other people's behaviour, but it is also key to *deception*.

◆ Deception is easily understood by the typical 4-year-old child. Whilst this may be socially discouraged, the fact that typical children understand deception and may attempt to deceive others is a sign of a normal ToM. This is because deception is nothing other than making someone else believe that

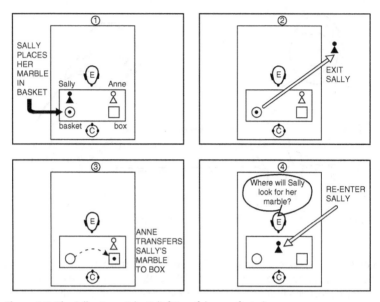

Figure 5.6 The Sally–Anne False Belief Test of theory of mind.
(C = Child; E = Experimenter)

something is true when in fact it is false. It is the process of manipulating another person's mind. Children with autism and Asperger syndrome are slow to understand deception, again a sign of a delay in the development of ToM. This means they are more at risk of being exploited for their gullibility. They tend to assume everyone is telling the truth, and may be shocked by the idea that other people may not say what they mean.

- The typical 6-year-old child is capable of understanding more complex (*second-order*) mindreading. In such tests based on the Sally–Anne false belief test, for example, Anne might peek back through a keyhole and see where Sally has moved her marble. Whilst the typical 6-year-old would have no trouble with this level of mindreading ('Sally *thinks* Anne doesn't *know* she has moved the marble'), children with autism and Asperger syndrome are again delayed in reaching this milestone.

- The typical 9-year-old child is capable of figuring out what might hurt another's feelings and what might therefore be better left unspoken, i.e. they can recognize *faux pas*. Children with Asperger syndrome are delayed by around 3 years in this skill, such that it is only when they are about 12 years old that they perform at the level of a typical 9-year-old, despite their normal IQ.

◈ While the typical 9-year-old can interpret another person's expressions from their eyes, to figure out what they might be thinking or feeling (see Figure 5.7), children with Asperger syndrome tend to find such tests far more difficult. The same is true when the adult test of *Reading the Mind in the Eyes* is used (Figure 5.8). Adults with autism and Asperger syndrome score below average on this test of *advanced* mindreading.

A strength of the mindblindness theory is that it can make sense of the social and communication difficulties in autism and Asperger syndrome, and that it is universal in applying to all individuals on the autistic spectrum. Its shortcoming is that it cannot account for the non-social features. A second limitation of this theory is that whilst mind *reading* is one component of empathy, empathy also requires an emotional response to another person's state of mind. Many people on the autistic spectrum also report that they are puzzled by how to *respond* to another person's emotions.

A final limitation of the mindblindness theory is that a range of clinical conditions show forms of mindblindness (such as patients with schizophrenia, or narcissistic and borderline personality disorders, and children with conduct disorder), so this may not be specific to autism and Asperger syndrome. This latter criticism of the theory is not so serious, since in these other conditions mindreading skills tend to be more preserved than in autism or Asperger Syndrome. For example, in schizophrenia, mindreading skills are preserved throughout childhood and adolescence and then become distorted with the onset of psychosis in young adulthood.

1. feeling sorry   2. bored

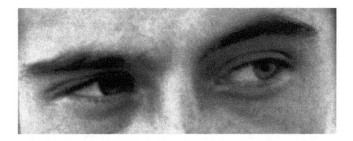

3. interested   4. joking

Figure 5.7 The child version of the *Reading the Mind in the Eyes Test.* Which word best describes what he is thinking or feeling? (Correct answer = interested).

1. sarcastic   2. stern

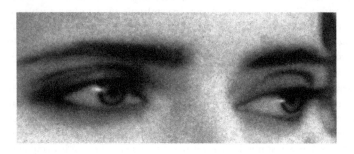

3. suspicious   4. dispirited

Figure 5.8 The adult version of the *Reading the Mind in the Eyes Test*. Which word best describes what she is thinking or feeling? (Correct answer = dispirited).

Two key ways to revise this theory have been to explain the non-social areas of strength by reference to a second factor, and to broaden the concept of ToM to include an emotional reactivity dimension. Both of these revisions were behind the development of the next theory.

The empathizing–systemizing theory

This theory explains the social and communication difficulties in autism and Asperger syndrome by reference to delays and deficits in *empathy*, whilst explaining the areas of strength by reference to intact or even superior skill in *systemizing*.

Empathy encompasses ToM or mindreading, but this is just the cognitive component of empathy (*cognitive empathy*). The second component of empathy is the response element: having an appropriate emotional reaction to another person's thoughts and feelings. This is referred to as the affective component of empathy (*affective empathy*).

On the Empathy Quotient (EQ), a questionnaire either filled out by an adult about themselves, or by a parent about their child, both cognitive and affective empathy are assessed. (There is a Child EQ, an Adolescent EQ, and an Adult EQ. See www.autismresearchcentre.com). Ten examples from the EQ are shown in Table 5.1.

If you agreed with items 1 and 3, this would get you two EQ points. If you disagreed with the remaining items, this would give you a total of 10 EQ points.

Table 5.1 The adult version of the Empathy Quotient (EQ): some examples

1.	I can easily tell if someone else wants to enter a conversation.
2.	I find it difficult to explain to others things that I understand easily, when they don't understand them first time.
3.	I really enjoy caring for other people.
4.	I find it hard to know what to do in a social situation.
5.	People often tell me that I went too far in driving my point home in a discussion.
6.	It doesn't bother me too much if I am late meeting a friend.
7.	Friendships and relationships are just too difficult, so I tend not to bother with them.
8.	I often find it difficult to judge if something is rude or polite.
9.	In a conversation, I tend to focus on my own thoughts rather than on what my listener might be thinking.
10.	When I was a child, I enjoyed cutting up worms to see what would happen.

In this case, the higher your score, the better your empathy. On this scale, people with autism spectrum conditions score lower than comparison groups.[1]

According to the empathizing–systemizing theory, autism and Asperger syndrome are best explained not just with reference to empathy (below average) but also with reference to a second psychological factor (systemizing), which is either average or even above average. So it is the *discrepancy* between E and S that determines if you are likely to develop autism or Asperger syndrome. To understand this theory better, we need to turn to the concept of *systemizing*.

Systemizing is the drive to analyse or construct systems. These might be any kind of system. What defines a system is that it follows *rules*, and when we systemize we are trying to identify the rules that govern the system, in order to predict how that system will behave. These are some of the major kinds of systems:

- *collectible* systems (e.g. distinguishing between types of stones)
- *mechanical* systems (e.g. a videorecorder or a window lock)
- *numerical* systems (e.g. a train timetable or a calendar)
- *abstract* systems (e.g. the syntax of a language or musical notation)
- *natural* systems (e.g. weather patterns or tidal wave patterns)
- *social* systems (e.g. a management hierarchy or a dance routine with a dance partner)
- *motoric* systems (e.g. throwing a Frisbee or bouncing on a trampoline).

In all these cases, you systemize by noting regularities (or structure) and rules. The rules tend to be derived by noting if A and B are *associated* in a systematic way (e.g. the musical note E is always five tones above the musical note A; or in 1995 the Car of the Year was a Fiat Punto). A second step in systemizing is to consider if the evidence allows you to conclude that A *causes* B (e.g. turning this electrical switch to the Up position causes this light to go on; or moving the Ayesha hydrangea from acidic to alkaline soil causes its colour to change from blue to pink).

The evidence for intact or even unusually strong systemizing in autism and Asperger syndrome is that such children performed above the level that one would expect on a physics test (see Figure 5.9). Children with Asperger syndrome as young as 8–11 years old scored higher than a comparison group who were older (typical teenagers).

A second piece of evidence comes from studies using the Systemizing Quotient (SQ). The SQ is another questionnaire that works in a very similar way to the EQ and AQ that we encountered earlier. You simply say if you agree or disagree with each statement as a description of you. (There is a Child SQ, an Adolescent SQ, and an Adult SQ. See http://www.autismresearchcentre.com). Table 5.2 lists 10 sample questions, each of which is asking you about how interested you are in different systems.

If you disagreed with items 5, 7 and 9 in Table 5.2, you would get 3 points on the SQ. If you agreed with the remaining items, that would earn you another 7 points on the SQ, making a total of 10. The higher your score, the stronger your drive to systemize. People with high-functioning autism or Asperger syndrome score higher on the SQ compared with people in the general population.

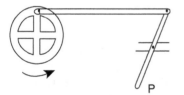

If the wheel rotates as shown, P will

(a) move to the right and top

(b) move to the left and top

(c) move to and fro

(d) none of these

Figure 5.9 The Intuitive Physics Test. (Correct answer = c)

Table 5.2 The adult version of the Systemizing Quotient-Revised (SQ-R): some examples

1.	I find it very easy to use train timetables, even if this involves several connections.
2.	I like music or book shops because they are clearly organized.
3.	When I read something, I always notice whether it is grammatically correct.
4.	I find myself categorizing people into types (in my own mind).
5.	I find it difficult to read and understand maps.
6.	When I look at a mountain, I think about how precisely it was formed.
7.	I am not interested in the details of exchange rates, interest rates, stocks and shares.
8.	If I were buying a car, I would want to obtain specific information about its engine capacity.
9.	I find it difficult to learn how to program video recorders.
10.	When I like something, I like to collect a lot of different examples of that type of object, so I can see how they differ from each other.

The above tests of systemizing are designed for children or adults with Asperger syndrome, not classic autism. However, children with classic autism perform better than controls on the *picture sequencing test* where the stories can be sequenced using physical–causal concepts. They also score above average on a test of how to figure out how a Polaroid camera works, even though they have difficulties figuring out people's thoughts and feelings. Both of these are signs of their intact or even strong systemizing[2].

The strength of the empathizing–systemizing theory is that it is a two-factor theory that can explain the cluster of both the social and non-social features in autism and Asperger syndrome. Below-average empathy is a way to explain the social communication difficulties, whilst average or even above-average systemizing is a way of explaining the narrow interests, repetitive behaviour and resistance to change/need for sameness. This is because when you systemize, it is essential to keep everything constant, and only vary one thing at a time. That way, you can see what might be causing what, rendering the world predictable. And to check if the pattern or rule you have identified is correct or consistent, it is essential to repeat the sequence over and over again.

When this theory first came out, one criticism of it was that it might only apply to the high-functioning individuals with autism or Asperger syndrome. Whilst their obsessions (with computers or maths, for example) could be seen in terms of strong systemizing, surely this didn't apply to the low-functioning individuals? However, when we think of a child with autism, many of the classic behaviours can be seen as a reflection of their strong systemizing. Some examples are listed here.

Systemizing in classic autism

- *Sensory systemizing*
    - Tapping surfaces, or letting sand run through one's fingers
    - Sniffing people, or eating the same food over and over again
- *Motoric systemizing*
    - Spinning round and round, or rocking back and forth
    - Flicking a straw at high speed in peripheral vision (stereotypies)
- *Collectable systemizing*
    - Collecting leaves or football stickers
    - Learning the flags of different countries
- *Numerical systemizing*
    - Obsessions with calendars or train timetables
    - Naming prime numbers, or memorizing birthdates or historical dates
- *Motion systemizing*
    - Watching washing machines spin round and round
    - Spinning the wheels of a toy car repeatedly
- *Spatial systemizing*
    - Naming shapes
    - Obsessions with routes
- *Environmental systemizing*
    - Insisting on toy bricks being lined up in an invariant order
    - Putting videos on the bookshelf in a strict order
- *Social systemizing*
    - Insisting on the same timetable at school
    - Saying the first half of a phrase or sentence and waiting for the other person to complete it

(continued)

Natural systemizing
  - Asking over and over again what the weather will be today
  - Classifying every dog

Mechanical systemizing
  - Learning to operate the VCR
  - Building Lego models

Vocal/auditory/verbal systemizing
  - Echoing sounds
  - Parroting sentences

Systemizing action sequences
  - Watching the same video over and over again
  - Repeating actions

Musical systemizing
  - Playing a tune on an instrument over and over again
  - Memorizing long sequences of musical notes

In contrast, a child with Asperger syndrome might show their strong systemizing rather differently.

Systemizing in Asperger syndrome

Sensory systemizing
  - Wearing the same clothes every day
  - Insisting on the same foods each day

Motoric systemizing
  - Practising skateboarding moves or frisbee moves
  - Learning knitting patterns

Collectible systemizing
  - Collecting the complete set of *Warhammer* or *Pokemon*
  - Making lists and catalogues

Numerical systemizing
  - Rapid calculation of prime numbers
  - Solving maths problems

(continued)

- *Motion systemizing*
  - Analysing exactly when a specific event occurs in a repeating cycle
  - Enjoying riding on merry-go-rounds

- *Spatial systemizing*
  - Studying maps
  - Developing drawing techniques

- *Environmental systemizing*
  - Knowing the names of the DVDs lined up on the bookshelf, in order
  - Insisting that nothing is moved from its usual position in the room

- *Social systemizing*
  - Learning the names and rank of every person in a battalion
  - Insisting on playing the same game whenever a child comes to play

- *Moral systemizing*
  - Insisting on other people following social rules
  - Becoming a whistle-blower

- *Natural systemizing*
  - Learning the names of every kind of tortoise
  - Learning the Latin names of every plant and their optimal growing conditions

- *Mechanical systemizing*
  - Taking the toaster apart and reassembling it
  - Fixing bicycles

- *Vocal/auditory/verbal systemizing*
  - Imitating accents
  - Collecting words and word meanings

- *Systemizing action sequences*
  - Watching the same movie dozens of times
  - Analysing dance techniques

- *Musical systemizing*
  - Mastering an instrument
  - Analysing the musical structure of a song

Just as a spider cannot help but spin webs — that is what they are evolved to do — so (according to this theory) the person with autism or Asperger syndrome just *has* to systemize everything. That is how their brain works. The content of their narrow interests reflects how they are strongly drawn to systemizable information.

Reconceptualizing repetitive behaviour and narrow interests in autism and Asperger syndrome

An advantage of the empathizing–systemizing theory is that it reconceptualizes the repetitive behaviour and narrow interests in people on the autistic spectrum. Whereas the executive dysfunction theory sees these as a sign of something in the brain being broken or undeveloped (the ability to shift and plan), and the weak central coherence theory sees these as a sign of something missing in the brain (the ability to integrate or perceive at the global level), the idea of strong systemizing sees these same behaviours as the result of intelligent behaviour (detailed analysis of systems, however small).

Reconceptualizing 'learning style' in autism spectrum conditions

Like the weak central coherence theory, the empathizing-systemizing theory is about a different *cognitive style* (a different style of thinking and learning). Like that theory, it also posits excellent attention to detail (in perception and memory), since when you systemize you have to pay attention to the tiny details. This is because each tiny detail in a system might have a functional role. In one cell phone, which is a mechanical/electronic system, one button may have a completely different function to the same button in a different make or model phone. In a mathematical calculation, changing one number in the sequence will totally change the workings of the system (the answer you get). So details matter.

The difference between these two theories is that whilst the weak central coherence theory sees people with autism spectrum conditions as drawn to detailed information (sometimes called local processing) for negative reasons (because of an alleged inability to integrate), the empathizing–systemizing theory sees this same quality (excellent attention to detail) as being highly purposeful: it is being done in order to understand a system. Attention to detail is occurring for positive reasons: it is *in the service* of achieving an ultimate understanding of a system (however small and specific that system might be).

The ultimate difference between these two theories is that whereas the weak central coherence theory predicts that people with autism or Asperger syndrome will be forever lost in the detail and never achieve an understanding of the system as a whole (since this would require a global overview), the empathizing–systemizing theory predicts that over time, the person can achieve an excellent understanding of a whole system, given the opportunity to observe and control all the variables in that system.

So, when the low-functioning person with classic autism has shaken that piece of string thousands of times close to his eyes, he knows exactly how the physics of that string movement works. He can make it move in exactly the same way every time. When he makes a long, rapid sequence of sounds, he knows exactly how that auditory system will work. When he picks up that Rubik's cube and goes through the same sequence of movements, he can reach the same outcome every time.

Reconceptualizing generalization difficulties in autism spectrum conditions

One final advantage of this theory is that it can explain what is sometimes seen as reduced generalization in autism or Asperger syndrome. It is sometimes said that people with autism or Asperger syndrome cannot generalize. You teach them about a specific car and you wait to see if they can generalize what they have learnt to all cars. You teach them how to go through a sequence of actions such as taking a shower in this particular bathroom at home, and you wait to see if they can generalize the sequence when you go to stay at granny's home, in a different bathroom. Often what is found is an inability to generalize.

According to the empathizing–systemizing theory, this is exactly what you would expect if the person is trying to understand each system as a unique system, since each system works slightly differently. For a strong systemizer, the differences between systems are of greater interest than their commonalities. If you treat all cars as the same, you miss out on discovering that one has features the other does not. Even if you lump all Renault Lagunas together, you miss out on understanding the difference between the dozens of different models of Renault Laguna. A good systemizer is a splitter, not a lumper, since lumping things together can lead to missing key differences that enable you to predict how these two things behave differently. Seen in this light, it is the neurotypical person who has a difficulty, skating over differences that might be very important. All that many neurotypical people see is that 'trees have leaves'. The person with autism sees every kind of tree having a totally different type of leaf, and even sees that within one type of tree (the Californian sycamore), some leaves on the sycamore tree have a fungal disease and some do not. Would you notice that?

So, if you are a strong systemizer, you only generalize to a specific system. You don't conclude that 'all computers are the same', when they are patently not. It would be a meaningless and superficial conclusion to draw. Sure, all computers process information, but how each type of computer works may be so completely different from another that it is next to worthless to focus on such a broad-brush overview. Premature generalizing is a sign of an unsystematic mind.

The extreme male brain theory

The empathizing–systemizing theory has been extended into the extreme male brain theory of autism. This is because there are clear sex differences in empathizing (females performing better on many tests of this) and in systemizing (males performing better on tests of this). Seen in this light, autism and Asperger syndrome can be conceptualized as an extreme of the typical male profile. This view was first put forward by the paediatrician Hans Asperger in 1944.

This theory is effectively just an extension of the empathizing–systemizing theory. That theory posits two independent dimensions, E (for empathy) and S (for systemizing), in which individual differences are observed in the population. When you plot these, five different 'brain types' are seen:

Brain types predicted by the empathizing–systemizing theory

- *Type E*
    - individuals whose empathy is stronger than their systemizing
    - denoted as E > S

- *Type S*
    - individuals whose systemizing is stronger than their empathy
    - denoted as S > E

(*continued*)

- *Type B* (for balanced)
    - individuals whose empathy is as good (or as bad) as their systemizing
    - denoted as $S = E$

- *Extreme Type E*
    - individuals whose empathy is above average, but who may be challenged when it comes to systemizing
    - denoted as $E \gg S$

- *Extreme Type S*
    - individuals whose systemizing is above average, but who may be challenged when it comes to empathy
    - denoted as $S \gg E$

Figure 5.10 shows the idealized model, which predicts that more females are likely to have a brain of Type E, and more males are likely to have a brain of Type S. People with autism spectrum conditions, if they are an extreme of the male brain, are predicted to be more likely to have a brain of Extreme Type S.

If one gives people in the general population measures of empathy and systemizing (the EQ and SQ), the results fit the above model reasonably well. Table 5.3 shows what percentage of males and females in the general population, and people with autism spectrum conditions, fall into each of the five main brain types. What can be seen is that more males do have a brain of Type S, more females have a brain of Type E, and the majority of people with autism and Asperger syndrome have an extreme of the male brain.

Looking at the same data graphically (Figure 5.11), one can see that more women fall into the Type E band, more men fall into the Type S band, and more people with autism spectrum conditions fall into the Extreme Type S band.

Apart from the evidence from the SQ and EQ, there is other evidence that supports the extreme male brain theory. Regarding tests of empathy, on the *faux pas test*, where a child has to recognize when someone has said something that could be hurtful, typically girls develop faster than boys, and children with autism spectrum conditions develop even more slowly than typical boys. On the *Reading the Mind in the Eyes Test*, where one has to decode subtle emotional expressions around a person's eyes, on average women score higher than men, and people with autism spectrum conditions score even lower than

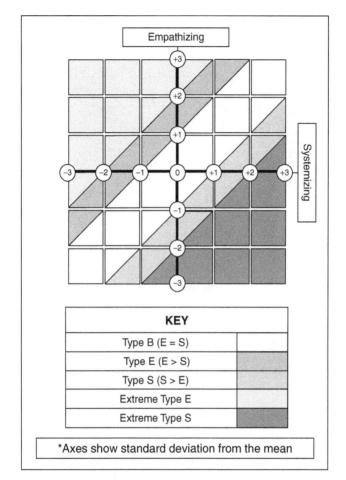

Figure 5.10 Modelling empathizing and systemizing, and the five 'brain types'.

Table 5.3 Percentage of people showing each of the three major brain types

Brain type	(Short-hand)	Men	Women	Asperger syndrome
E > S	Female brain	17	44	1
S > E	Male brain	54	17	27
S >> E	Extreme male	6	0	65

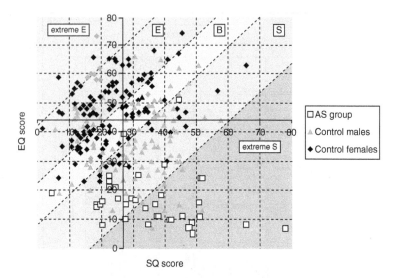

Figure 5.11 EQ and SQ scores broadly match predictions from the extreme male brain theory. AS = Asperger syndrome.

typical males. Regarding tests of attention to detail, on the *Embedded Figures Test* where one has to find a target shape as quickly as possible, on average males are faster than females, and people with autism are even faster than typical males.

Recently, the extreme male brain theory has been extended to the level of neurology, with some interesting findings emerging. Thus, in some regions of the brain that on average are smaller in males than in females, people with autism have even smaller brain regions than typical males. In contrast, in some regions of the brain that on average are bigger in males than in females, people with autism have even bigger brain regions than typical males. (These generalizations are not clear-cut because they depend on the timing in development). Also, the male brain on average is larger than in females, and people with autism have been found to have even larger brains than typical males. Not all studies support this pattern, but some do, and it will be important to study such patterns further. Some of these regions are listed in the boxes below.

Regions of the brain that are smaller in males than females, and in autism are even smaller than in typical males

- Anterior cingulate

- Superior temporal gyrus

- Inferior frontal gyrus

Regions of the brain that are bigger in males than females, and in autism are even bigger than in typical males

- Amygdala (in early life)

- Overall brain size/weight

- Head circumference

Using a measure called the 2D:4D ratio (the ratio between the length of the second and the fourth finger), it has been found that this is lower in typical males than typical females, and in autism this is even smaller than in typical males. This is thought to be a reflection of prenatal testosterone levels. We return to these neurobiological findings in Chapter 6, but again this finding fits the idea of autism being an extreme of the male brain. In summary, the extreme male brain theory is a relatively new theory that may be important for understanding why more males develop autism and Asperger syndrome than do females. It remains in need of further examination.

The magnocellular theory

A new theory of autism suggests that there is a specific dysfunction in one visual pathway in the brain (the magnocellular pathway) that is responsible for processing motion, whilst the other major pathway (the parvocellular pathway) is intact. Some evidence for this theory is that on the flicker pedestal test, where one is presented with 4 squares that appear, one at a time, at a rapid speed, and one has to say when a new square appears, people with autism are reported to be slower to respond to such change. This is an important new theory because it makes testable predictions at the cellular and neuronal level. It is included as a psychological theory because currently it has only been tested using psychological methods.

One potential problem for this theory is that it suggests a purely visual difficulty, whereas sensory issues in autism (hypersensitivity) appear to be a feature of all senses. This theory also predicts that people with autism will avoid moving or changing stimuli because they cannot process them, whereas in fact children with autism become strongly attracted to objects that move in predictable patterns (such as objects that spin: washing machines, toy car wheels, electric fans, etc.). Another potential problem for this theory is that magnocellular abnormalities have been found in other conditions (including dyslexia), so it is unclear if it can account for the specific profile seen in autism and Asperger syndrome. A final problem for this theory is that in an auditory equivalent of the flicker test, people with autism are *quicker* to detect the change. Resolving such contradictions between results will be important for research in the future. The potential value of this theory is that this theory is simultaneously a psychological and a neurological theory and opens up new questions for research.

Summary and comparison of the five theories

We have reviewed the five major psychological theories of autism and Asperger syndrome. These are:

- Executive dysfunction theory
- Weak central coherence theory
- Mindblindness theory
- Empathizing–systemizing theory
    - and by extension, the extreme male brain theory
- Magnocellular theory

It may be confusing for some people to understand why different psychological theories have been proposed, why the differences between them matter, how these might develop in future years, and how theories can be tested. The easiest way of explaining how to evaluate different theories is to keep in mind what such theories are put forward to explain. There is a wide array of behaviours in autism and Asperger syndrome, and the purpose of a theory is to reduce this array to one or several underlying causal factors. Table 5.4 lists the array of behaviours to be explained, and shows which behaviours each of the five major theories can explain.

Table 5.4 Which behaviours each of the five psychological theories can explain

Features to be explained	Domain	WCC	EF	ToM	Magnocellular	E-S/ EMB
Hand flapping	Motor		√			√
Tip-toe walking	Motor					
Non-right-handedness	Motor					√
Dyspraxia	Motor	√	√			
Love of rule-governed fictional worlds	Repetition			√		√
Stereotypies and twiddling	Repetition		√			√
Wearing the same clothes every day	Repetition		√			√
Insisting on the same foods each day	Repetition		√			√
Watching the same movie multiple times	Repetition			√		

(continued)

Key : √ = can be explained by the theory; WCC = Weak Central Coherence theory; EF = Executive Function theory; ToM = Theory of Mind/Mindblindness; E-S = Empathizing-Systemizing theory; EMB = Extreme Male Brain theory

Table 5.4 Which behaviours each of the five psychological theories can explain (*continued*)

Features to be explained	Domain	WCC	EF	ToM	Magnocellular	E-S/ EMB
Routines and rituals	Repetition		√			√
Enjoyment of games with repetitive techniques/rules	Repetition		√			√
Tantrums over change or other points of view	Repetition		√	√		√
Obsessions with systems, narrow interests	Repetition	√				√
Preference for rules and patterns	Repetition					√
Creating systems and order	Repetition					√
Love of repetition	Repetition		√			√
Rigid behaviour	Repetition		√			√
Hyper-control	Repetition					√
Syntactic talent	Language/ communication					√
Too much detail in communication (inability to edit)	Language/ communication		√			√
Literal language	Language/ communication			√		√
Delays in protodeclarative pointing	Language/ communication			√		√

(*continued*)

Table 5.4 Which behaviours each of the five psychological theories can explain (*continued*)

Features to be explained	Domain	WCC	EF	ToM	Magnocellular	E-S/ EMB
Too little information in answers	Language/ communication			√		√
Language delay	Language/ communication			√		√
Echolalia	Language/ communication			√		√
Poor at pragmatics	Language/ communication			√		√
Pronoun reversal	Language/ communication			√		√
Difficulties with figurative language, including jokes	Language/ communication			√		√
Precocious vocabulary	Language/ communication					√
Delay in joint attention (including gaze monitoring)	Social			√		√
Self-centredness (me, me, me)	Social			√		√
Preference for adult company	Social			√		√
Lack of self-awareness	Social			√		√
Insisting on own desires	Social			√		√
Bossy, controlling behaviour	Social			√		√

(*continued*)

Table 5.4 Which behaviours each of the five psychological theories can explain (*continued*)

Features to be explained	Domain	WCC	EF	ToM	Magnocellular	E-S/ EMB
Understanding deception	Social			√		√
Preference for solitude	Social			√		√
No diplomacy or white lies	Social			√		√
Poor at anticipating the consequences of own actions on others' feelings	Social		√	√		√
Difficulty in coping in social groups (more than 1 to 1)	Social			√		√
Insisting on others following rules	Social			√		√
Becoming a whistle-blower	Social			√		√
Difficulty reading emotions/ intentions	Social			√		√
Frequent *faux pas*	Social		√	√		√
Difficulties perceiving biological motion	Social			√	√	√
No interest in pretend play	Social			√		√
Easily duped/ gullible	Social			√		√
Unusual eye contact	Social			√	√	√

(continued)

Table 5.4 Which behaviours each of the five psychological theories can explain *(continued)*

Features to be explained	Domain	WCC	EF	ToM	Magnocellular	E-S/ EMB
Difficulties with emotion recognition	Social			√		√
Morality based on laws of justice rather than affect	Social			√		√
Difficulty seeing other's perspective	Social			√		√
Tendency towards monologue	Social		√	√		√
Difficulties turn-taking	Social		√	√		√
Intrusion into personal space	Social			√		√
Lack of reciprocity and poor social skills	Social	√		√		√
Can't see the point of pretending	Social			√		√
Delay in passing false belief	Social			√		√
Sex differences in typical cognition	Cognition					√
No interest in estimation or approximation	Cognition					√
Truth-seeking	Cognition					√
Bigger picture planning difficulties	Cognition	√	√			√

(continued)

Table 5.4 Which behaviours each of the five psychological theories can explain (*continued*)

Features to be explained	Domain	WCC	EF	ToM	Magnocellular	E-S/ EMB
Monotropism	Cognition		√			√
Local processing	Cognition	√				√
Reluctance to generalize	Cognition					√
Intact intuitive physics	Cognition			√		√
Intact reasoning	Cognition			√		√
Musical talent	Cognition					√
Islets of ability in art, memory, calculation	Cognition					√
Precision and exactness, an eye for detail	Cognition		√			√
Doing one thing at a time/difficulty multitasking	Cognition		√			√
Good memory for details/facts	Cognition		√			√
Black and white thinking	Cognition			√		√
Collecting the complete set	Cognition		√			√
Learning lists of names/ events/facts	Cognition					√
Making lists	Cognition					√
Cataloguing/ classifying	Cognition					√

(*continued*)

Table 5.4 Which behaviours each of the five psychological theories can explain *(continued)*

Features to be explained	Domain	WCC	EF	ToM	Magnocellular	E-S/ EMB
Collecting word meanings	Cognition					√
Error-checking	Cognition					√
Counting	Cognition					√
Solving maths problems	Cognition					√
Memorizing calendars, timetables	Cognition					√
Risk of reduced IQ	Cognition	√	√			?
Understanding a whole system	Cognition					√
Superiority on the Block Design Test	Cognition	√				√
Superior attention to detail	Cognition	√				√
Sensory hypersensitivity	Cognition	√				√
Good at jigsaw puzzles	Cognition	√				√
Difficulties with attention shifting	Cognition		√			√
Interest in science-fiction but not pure fiction	Cognition			√		√
Hyperlexia	Cognition					√
Low spatial frequency	Cognition				√	

WCC = weak cental coherence; EF = executive dysfunction; ToM = theory of mind; E-S/EMB = Empathizing–systemizing/extreme male brain.

From the list in Table 5.4, it is apparent that the empathizing–systemizing theory can explain more characteristics of autism and Asperger syndrome than the other four theories. Table 5.4 should be read as a reminder to theorists as to what needs to explained. There is a danger that theories are put forward that explain one corner of autism or Asperger syndrome, but not the whole spectrum. Psychological theories of the autistic spectrum need to explain the breadth of the spectrum. The hope is that in the future, such theories will become integrated with the neurobiology of autism and Asperger syndrome, reviewed next.

6

The biology of autism and Asperger syndrome

→ Key points

There is no longer any doubt that autism spectrum conditions are biological in orgin. The strongest evidence supports the genetic theory. Heritability of autism and Asperger syndrome is not 100 per cent. This means there must be some environmental component too, in all likelihood interacting with the risk genes. We do not yet know what the environmental factors are. There is not yet a biological marker with which to diagnose autism spectrum conditions, but research into the biomedical aspects is being accelerated. Evidence points to atypical brain development pre- and post-natally, particularly affecting processing of social information.

In Chapter 1 we heard that in 1964 Bruno Bettelheim suggested that autism was due to purely *emotional* consequences of insufficient parental affection. Even as late as 1982, when Niko Tinbergen wrote his book describing *anxiety* as a cause of autism, it was still possible to maintain that this syndrome was due to purely *psychogenic* factors. Psychogenic means purely 'in the mind'; as if the mind had no connection with the brain and as if we were dealing with a child with a normally developing brain whose emotions were the only aspect that was in some way failing to develop normally.

Theories suggesting that autism is caused by purely psychological factors[1] have been refuted by a large body of biomedical research revealing a large set of differences in the autistic brain. This chapter summarizes what we know about the biology of autism and Asperger syndrome.

A major tool that has enabled scientists to study the autistic brain, whilst the person is alive, has been brain scanning (Figure 6.1), and this has changed across the decades. In the 1970s it was fashionable to use CT (computerized tomography) scans, in the 1980s SPECT (single-photon emission computerized tomography), in the 1990s PET (positron emission tomography) and in the twenty-first century MRI (magnetic resonance imaging). What have we learnt?

Overall brain volume and growth

The most striking finding is that children with autism go through a period of *brain overgrowth* in the first few years of life, i.e. their head (and brain) is growing at a faster rate than average. This is evident in measures of *head*

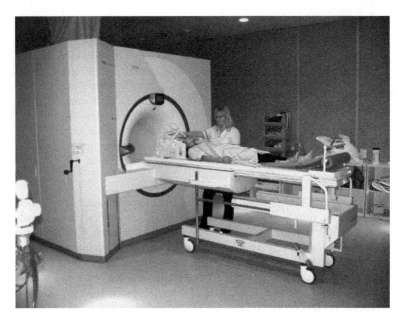

Figure 6.1 An MRI scanner.

circumference (if you measure this with a tape measure around the skull), but it is also evident using structural brain scanning (which provides a snapshot of the size of the brain at a single point in development). It is also evident at post-mortem where studies have discovered the brain is both bigger and heavier in autism. These differences do not apply to every individual with a diagnosis, but become apparent when two groups (those with a diagnosis and those without) are compared. So these are differences on average.

Quite what is causing the accelerated brain development and early overgrowth is unclear. Post-mortem studies suggest that there is increased cell density (more neurons or nerve cells) in regions of the brain such as the *hippocampus* and *amygdala*, as well as more *dendrites* (or connections between neurons). There is also more generalized overgrowth (hyperplasia), especially in the frontal lobes. Other studies however find the opposite abnormality: fewer neurons in the amygdala for example. Further research is needed into these differences.

Differences in brain structure

When different regions of the brain are compared, certain regions show more differences than others. Thus, a consistent finding is that the *amygdala* (involved in emotional responses and recognizing emotions in others), the *hippocampus* (involved in memory), the *caudate nucleus* and parts of the *cerebellum* (involved in attention switching and coordination) are smaller, in autism. However, the amygdala is smaller than average in adolescents and adults with autism, whilst the amygdala is larger than average in younger children with autism. A subgroup of people with autism have an abnormally large cerebellum.

In addition, there is more *grey matter* and *white matter* in the autistic brain, especially in the frontal lobes (particularly in the dorsolateral prefrontal and medial prefrontal cortex). Grey matter mostly contains the cell bodies of nerve cells, whilst white matter mostly contains their axons (or connections). A simple way to understand the difference is that grey matter is involved in the neuronal computation whilst white matter is involved in carrying the information. Some studies suggest that this overgrowth of grey matter is only found in early development (before 5 years old) and not after. Further studies will be needed to confirm this developmental pattern. Early increases in grey matter could reflect the presence of too many nerve cells.

Differences in brain function

SPECT, PET and functional MRI (fMRI) allow not just a snapshot of brain structure but images of brain activity whilst the person is engaged in a task of some kind. The activity that is recorded is usually *oxygenated blood flow*, and the assumption that neuroscientists make is that if oxygenated blood flow is greater in one region in the brain whilst the person is engaged in a task (such as looking at upright faces) compared with when they are engaged in a control task (such as looking at inverted faces), then that region of the brain must be involved in performing that task (e.g. looking at upright faces). This is because more oxygenated blood would be required to support the 'work' being done in that brain region. Increases or decreases in oxygenated blood flow during a task in different brain regions are therefore taken as a proxy for differences in brain function—in how the brain works when it is trying to solve a task.

What has been found is that when people with autism are engaged in *mind-reading* tasks (thinking about other people's thoughts, feelings, intentions or emotions), a network of regions that for shorthand form what is called the *social brain* is consistently underactive in people with autism. This network includes at least seven brain regions:

Regions in the social brain

- Medial prefrontal cortex

- Orbito-frontal cortex

- Amygdala

- Fusiform face area

- Temporal–parietal junction

- Superior temporal gyrus

- Inferior frontal gyrus

- Anterior cingulate cortex

- Posterior cingulate cortex/precuneus

Each of these regions is activated during different aspects of empathy or mindreading, in the typical brain, and is underactive in the autistic brain. Figure 6.2 shows the schematic location of each of these brain regions.

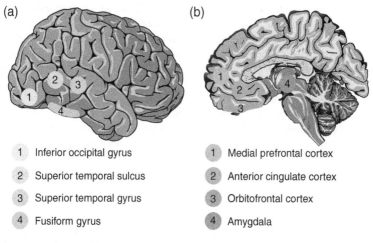

1 Inferior occipital gyrus

2 Superior temporal sulcus

3 Superior temporal gyrus

4 Fusiform gyrus

1 Medial prefrontal cortex

2 Anterior cingulate cortex

3 Orbitofrontal cortex

4 Amygdala

Figure 6.2 The social brain.

The mirror neuron theory

One new neurobiological theory to emerge in recent years has been called the 'mirror neuron' theory of autism. The idea is that in the typical brain, certain regions are active not only when the person themselves performs an action (e.g. reaching for a cup) but also when that person observes another person performing the same action (e.g. reaching for a cup).

The *mirror neuron* theory first emerged from animal research (using monkeys): when a deep electrode was implanted into the brain to measure the electrical activity of particular nerve cells (or assemblies of nerve cells), the very same cells fired both when performing an action and when perceiving another animal performing that action. In monkeys, these mirror neurons are in the ventral premotor cortex (which in humans is probably equivalent to the inferior frontal gyrus) and in the inferior parietal lobe.

However, whereas it is possible to study individual neurons (or clusters of these) in animals, it is not yet possible to image individual neurons in humans. So, the term 'mirror neuron' is something of a misnomer. Calling it a 'mirror system' may be slightly more accurate. Despite this terminological point, the idea of a mirror system in the brain is potentially very important, as it may explain how we learn from others, how we identify with others and how we make sense of others' behaviour (i.e., how we become social).

Neuroimaging studies have found that when children with autism *make* facial expressions of emotion, or *look* at someone else's facial expression of emotion, they show less activity in the *pars opercularis* relative to the typically developing child's brain. The pars opercularis is a part of the inferior frontal gyrus. It is thought to be part of the mirror system, leading to the idea that autism is a syndrome involving a 'broken mirror'. Leaving aside this unfortunate metaphor, the neuroscience behind it is potentially important. However, it should be noted that there is one fact that does not fit the theory: namely, that some people with autism have excellent imitation skills in some areas (such as echolalia, or echoing another person's speech, and even their accent and intonation with great exactness).

Differences in neurotransmitter levels

Brain structure and blood flow are not the only differences that emerge in studies of the autistic brain. In addition, neurotransmitters (chemicals involved in carrying the electrochemical message or signal from one neuron to another, enabling the signal to jump across the synapse or gap between neurons) have been found to differ. Two key neurotransmitters that show altered levels are *serotonin* (also known as 5-hydroxytryptamine, or 5-HT) and *GABA* (γ-aminobutyric acid).

Serotonin

Serotonin is a monoamine neurotransmitter, synthesized in the serotonergic neurons in the central nervous system, as well as in the gastrointestinal tract. It plays an important role in regulating anger, aggression, mood, sleep and appetite. Its name reflects how it was discovered. (Serotonin means 'affecting blood vessel tone', since it was originally found to constrict vascular tone.) Its chemical name (5-HT) is often used instead.

A range of psychiatric conditions have *low* levels of serotonin, including depression and obsessive–compulsive disorder (OCD), as measured in peripheral blood. In a proportion of people with autism, however, the abnormality is the opposite: *elevated* levels of serotonin. It is unclear what effects these elevated levels of serotonin may have in autism.

GABA

GABA is produced by GABAergic neurons. GABA has an inhibitory role in the adult brain, so finding reduced levels of GABA is of interest in that it might leave the person with autism in an over-responsive, overstimulated state.

This might be very relevant to the anxiety and sensory hypersensitivity in autism. In mammalian development, GABA may have excitatory effects, which again could leave the individual feeling overwhelmed by too much neuronal firing.

Differences in electrophysiology

A different way of studying brain function is to measure electrical activity on the scalp, using *EEGs* (electroencephalograms) or the closely related method of *ERP* (event-related potentials). These involve putting electrodes onto the scalp that detect electrical activity across the surface of the skull, but emanating from different points within the brain. Whilst EEG tends to be used to measure the brain 'at rest' and is often used in the diagnosis of epilepsy, ERP is used to measure the speed with which the brain detects a stimulus (visual or auditory, usually) when the stimulus is presented. These electrophysiological methods are considered to be superior to other forms of brain scanning (PET, fMRI) in terms of temporal resolution, but inferior in terms of spatial localization (not being able to narrow down where in the brain the electrical signal is coming from).

Using ERP, it has been found that the *P3a,* also called the 'novelty P3' (the electrical wave seen whenever you hear a novel sound in a sequence of repetitive sounds) is inconsistent in autism. It is assumed that to detect novelty you need to switch attention, and that this might therefore indicate that a smaller shift of attention is occurring in autism. However, all we can really say is that this is an indicator of atypical attention. Given the findings that people with autism have heightened sensory sensitivity, it may simply mean that their brain only has to make a small shift in attention to detect fine differences.

ERP has been used not only with auditory stimuli but also with visual stimuli. For example, the *N170* in the typical brain is larger when presented with faces than with non-faces, especially in the right hemisphere. But in children with autism, the N170 (in one study) was larger for furniture than for faces, on both sides of their brain. These findings demonstrate that electrophysiological methods are sensitive to the atypical functioning of the 'social brain' in autism.

Evidence from post-mortem studies

Brain scanning methods are quite blunt instruments for looking at the fine-grained differences between the autistic and the typical brain. Brain scanning does not yet allow one to image individual cells in the brain. In contrast, the traditional methods of post-mortem histopathology can do this, though of course such science is slowed down by the availability of such tissue for research. From the autistic brains that have been studied at post-mortem it has emerged that there are fewer *Purkinje cells* in the cerebellum. This has been replicated in several different studies.

Purkinje cells are GABAergic neurons located in the cerebellum, with a large number of dendritic spines (branches between neurons). They have inhibitory functions and have a central role in co-ordination. The other key finding to have emerged from post-mortem neuropathology is increased cell density, increased packing of neurons and smaller cell size, in the hippocampus, amygdala, anterior cingulate, entorhinal cortex and mammillary bodies. These are all in the *limbic system* of the brain.

The amygdala abnormalities have given rise to an *amygdala theory of autism*, linked to the *Klüver–Bucy syndrome*. In this syndrome, artificially created in the laboratory, a monkey's amgydalae (both of them, one on each side of the brain) are lesioned (experimentally destroyed). The monkey reacts by becoming socially withdrawn, having difficulties recognizing if another monkey is friendly or aggressive, becoming hyperoral (putting everything into its mouth), socially disinhibited and even showing repetitive behaviours. For this reason, the Klüver–Bucy syndrome has been taken as a possible animal model of autism.

This certainly highlights the importance of the amygdala as a key structure in the 'social brain'. We should remember that a true animal model of autism may not be possible, given that autism also involves difficulties in communication and empathy, which are far more elaborate in humans.

Evidence for genetic factors

There is no longer any doubt that autism and Asperger syndrome are heritable conditions, meaning that genes inherited from one or both parents play a causal role in the development of the autistic brain. We can say this with certainty because of:

> * *Twin studies*: if one twin has autism, the chances of the co-twin also having an ASC is much higher (60–90 per cent) in identical (monozygotic twins) than non-identical (dizygotic twins), where the chance of them both having it (the concordance rate) is only about 5–10 per cent.
>
> * *Autism runs in families*: if there is one child in the family with autism or Asperger syndrome, the chances of another sibling also having an autism spectrum condition is about 5–10 per cent.
>
> (*continued*)

> * *Related conditions run in families*: other siblings may not have autism or Asperger syndrome but may have a related developmental condition, such as dyslexia or delayed language.
>
> * *The Broader Autism Phenotype*: parents and siblings (who are first-degree relatives) show mild echoes of autism, sometimes referred to as the Broader Autism Phenotype (BAP). This might take the form of being socially withdrawn or confused by social interaction, or mildly obsessive (in the sense of having strong narrow interests or a need for sameness) or having excellent attention to detail and remarkable memory. Although they don't have autism or Asperger sydrome itself, they have a milder manifestation of the same characteristics.
>
> * *Chromosomal abnormalities* (such as deletions or duplications) have been found, for example, on chromosome 15q11–q13.
>
> * *Mutations or variations in candidate genes* have been found to differ between people with autism spectrum conditions and typical individuals. Some of the genes include the *FOXP2*, *RAY1/ST7*, *IMMP2L* and *RELN* genes at 7q22–q33, the $GABA_A$ receptor subunit and *UBE3A* genes on chromosome 15q11–q13, the serotonin transporter gene (*5-HTT*) on 17q11–q12 and the oxytocin receptor gene at 3p25–p26. [The string of numbers and letters indicates the chromosome number that the gene is on, like an address.]

It is not yet known how many risk (or 'susceptibility') genes an individual needs to have in order to develop autism or Asperger syndrome, or what the genetic differences are between these two subgroups, and as yet there is no single gene or set of genes that is diagnostic of autism spectrum conditions.

Evidence for steroid hormonal factors

Surprisingly, given that autism and Asperger syndrome affect males far more often than females, it is strange that there has not been more research into the role of sex-related hormones (the steroid hormones) such as *testosterone* (and other androgens), or *oestrogen*.

Androgens is the generic term for steroid hormones which control masculinization of the body and the brain in all vertebrates. They work by binding to *androgen receptors* that are found all over the body and particularly in the brain. There is only one type of androgen receptor. Androgens come from the testes in males, and from the adrenal glands in both males and females. Hence males usually have much higher levels of testosterone.

93

One part of the adrenal gland (the *zona reticularis*) produces androgens from cholesterol, synthesizing, for example, DHEA (dehydroepiandrosterone) and androstenedione. These are 'weaker' steroids, compared with the potent hormone, testosterone. For example, androstenedione is said to be seven times weaker than testosterone in its masculinizing effects. Some cancers, such as prostate cancer, are hormone sensitive, in that they need testosterone to grow. For this reason, such cancers are treated with hormone therapy.

Oestrogens are also steroid hormones, and bind to oestrogen receptors. There are two types of oestrogen receptor, called α and β, and it is the β receptor that is of interest since these are found in the brain. The three types of oestrogens are called oestradiol, oestriol and oestrone. Although most people think androgens and oestrogens are quite different, in fact oestrogens are produced from androgens, converted through the action of enzymes (such as aromatase). For example, testosterone (an androgen) is converted by aromatase into oestradiol. So the so-called male and female hormones are in fact closely related.

When oestrogens are found in plants (such as soya or clover), these are called phyto-oestrogens. Oestrogens are produced in the ovary in females, but also by the adrenal glands in both sexes. Hence females have much higher levels of oestrogens. Many breast cancers are hormone sensitive in that they need oestrogen to grow. For this reason, such cancers are treated by hormone therapy, also known as anti-oestrogen therapy.

This is relevant to autism in that one Dutch study found that boys with autism were more likely to reach puberty earlier than average. Timing of puberty in males is in part regulated by testosterone levels. A British study found that women with Asperger syndrome were more likely to reach puberty later than average (only delayed by about 9 months), as indexed by the first menstrual period, known as *menarche*. Timing of puberty in girls is influenced by oestrogen and testosterone levels.

Women with Asperger syndrome are also more likely to have had *polycystic ovary syndrome* (PCOS). This is diagnosed when a woman has irregular menstrual cycles, delayed menarche and excess hirsutism (body hair), all signs that can be the consequence of high levels of testosterone. They also have higher rates of breast and ovarian cancer, which again are hormone sensitive. It is of interest that these same features (elevated rates of PCOS and of hormone-sensitive cancers) are also seen in mothers of children with autism. This is indirect evidence for hormonal dysregulation, presumably stemming from genetic factors.

The idea that hormonal factors may play a part in autism and Asperger syndrome is relevant to the *foetal androgen theory* of autism. Foetal testosterone is known to masculinize the brain in other animals. Studies have followed women who had amniocentesis during pregnancy (a routine clinical procedure in which the amniotic fluid in which the baby is bathed is extracted using a long needle, and which can be analysed for testosterone secreted by the foetus). When the children were followed-up after birth, those children with higher levels of foetal testosterone had lower rates of eye contact and were slower to develop language, as toddlers. In primary school they had more social difficulties and reduced empathy, and they also had stronger interests in systemizing.

These studies looked at individual differences in otherwise typically developing children. We cannot yet conclude that elevated rates of foetal testosterone cause autism or Asperger syndrome, as the children in these studies do not have a diagnosis. It is of interest that using the Child AQ (Autism Spectrum Quotient), mentioned in Chapter 3, completed by the mother, those children with higher levels of foetal testosterone also had a higher score on the AQ (more autistic traits). But the test of the foetal androgen theory will come when large enough samples of amniotic fluid are available, with follow-up data relating to actual diagnosis.

Evidence for peptide hormone factors

There are two non-steroid hormones that have become linked to autism over the years. These are both peptide hormones.

The first is *oxytocin*, of interest because it can act as a neurotransmitter in the brain. Oxytocin levels are below average in autism. Oxytocin is sometimes referred to as the 'social peptide' because it plays a key role in social relationships. This includes childbirth (oxytocin is released in women after distension of the cervix and vagina during labour, triggering the birth process), attachment (oxytocin is released in women after stimulation of the nipples during breastfeeding, triggering the 'let down' reflex in lactation) and romantic intimacy (oxytocin is released in both sexes during orgasm). Oxytocin levels, measured in the blood plasma, are highest in humans when they report they are falling in love.

Oxytocin is made in the magnocellular neurosecretory cells in the hypothalamus of the brain and then released into the blood from the pituitary gland. Oxytocin differs from another peptide hormone, called *vasopressin*, by only two amino acids. Oxytocin needs to bind to oxytocin receptors to become active. There are large numbers of oxytocin receptors in regions of the brain such as the amygdala and ventromedial prefrontal cortex, both regions that are underactive in autism, during certain kinds of social stimulation.

Oxytocin first came to attention as playing a key role in social behaviour following the study of two species of vole (a small mouse-like animal). The male prairie vole is completely faithful to his female mate, because of the oxytocin released into her brain and vasopressin released into his brain during sex. In contrast, the male meadow vole (a closely related species) is highly promiscuous. When a single gene controlling oxytocin is spliced, scientists demonstrated that the meadow vole's promiscuity reduces and he becomes more like a prairie vole. From living a socially isolated life, only getting together to mate, he moves into a more sociable lifestyle, living in the family and caring for young offspring.

Human studies have also shown that if a person's oxytocin levels are boosted (e.g. using a nasal spray of oxytocin), their ability to recognize emotional expressions in others' faces improves, as does their memory for faces, and they show more trust in their interactions (in a game where one has to anticipate how another person might behave). Intravenous infusions of oxytocin in autism have also been found to increase emotion-recognition skills.

It is not yet clear if oxytocin as a pharmacological treatment will have specific effects just on social behaviour and empathy since when oxytocin is given to people with autism, there are reports of reductions in the amount of repetitive behaviour. This may mean that it is also reducing systemizing. More research will be needed into this interesting hormone. Potential side-effects could include increased erections in males, since oxytocin injections in rats have this consequence. Note that one of the genetic findings that has been replicated in autism is that a variant of the oxytocin receptor gene is more frequent in autism than in controls.

No credible evidence for vaccination damage

In 1997, a London-based doctor, Andrew Wakefield, and his team, published an article in the leading medical journal the *Lancet*. They suggested that autism may be caused by the MMR vaccine (against measles, mumps and rubella viruses). This was based on a study of 12 children. As a result of this article and the media frenzy that published alarmist stories, parental uptake of the MMR (triple) vaccination dropped as low as 60 per cent, well below the level of 95 per cent required to provide 'herd immunity'. This posed real public health concerns because for the first time in a decade, cases of measles were reported across Britain, and measles can be potentially fatal.

The evidence against the MMR theory of autism is that in a study of more than 30 000 children in Japan, where the MMR triple vaccine was withdrawn, cases of autism continued to rise (see Figure 6.3). In Denmark, where it was possible to compare two large populations (those who had had MMR when it was introduced and those who had not had MMR because it was not yet introduced), rates of autism did not differ. These two findings thus suggest there is no evidence to link MMR with autism. Media reporting has been criticized (e.g. *Daily Mail*, 22 March 2006 with the headlines 'MMR fears coming true') as contributing to the public misinformation on science.

Most of Andrew Wakefield's co-authors on the *Lancet* article have now publicly stated that they wish to retract their claim, and Wakefield was asked to resign his position at the Royal Free Hospital in London because it could be argued that in clinging to a theory for which there was no strong evidence and which could potentially do harm (to the public health vaccination programme), he was potentially in breach of the Hippocratic oath governing medical practice ('do no harm'). He has since gone to work in Texas, supported by the pro-MMR lobby group, since a percentage of parents remain convinced that MMR damaged their child's brain. This may reflect the need in parents to attach the 'blame' to someone or something in the environment.

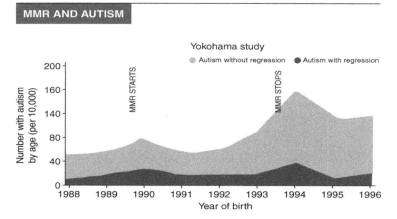

Figure 6.3 MMR and autism.

Differences in rates of associated conditions

It has long been known that autism is associated with other conditions, some of which are of neurological origin. These include (but are not restricted to) the following.

Psychiatric conditions

* *Depression*: found in at least 50 per cent of people with Asperger syndrome, partially because of their greater awareness of being different and greater awareness of their difficulties.

* *Anxiety*: particularly social anxiety.

* *Obsessive–compulsive disorder (OCD)*: this should not be confused with the 'obsessions' that are part of autism, but which are really just narrow interests. In OCD, the term 'obsession' refers to intrusive thoughts that cause anxiety.

* *Anorexia*: some studies suggest this may be undiagnosed Asperger syndrome in girls, involving a narrow interest that happens to focus on weight and food intake, but which may be part of a picture of social difficulties.

* *Psychosis and schizophrenia*: these are rare but very serious, requiring anti-psychotic medication.

Cognitive and learning disabilities

* *Attention deficit and hyperactivity disorder (ADHD)*: A subgroup of people on the autistic spectrum also have ADHD. Another subgroup of people with autism and Asperger Syndrome have the opposite profile: an excellent ability to concentrate on one topic for extended periods.

* *Learning difficulties*: this used to be said to be as high as 75 per cent of people with autism but today is thought to be much lower, possibly only 25 per cent.

Medical conditions

- *Neuroinflammation and immune disorders*: these include asthma and eczma.

- *Gastrointestinal (GI) tract problems*: e.g. irritable bowel syndrome apparently found in as many as 50 per cent of people on the autistic spectrum.

- *Epilepsy*: this can be relatively late onset, such as during adolescence. The presence of epilepsy was originally one of the strongest clues that autism was a neurodevelopmental condition.

- *Fragile X syndrome*: in which a part of the X chromosome is expanded in up to 4% of people with autism. This leads to an absence of Fragile X Mental Retardation Protein (FMRP), causing runaway 'plasticity' among neurons.

- *Tuberous sclerosis (TS)*: this involves benign tumours growing in the body and in the brain. Fifty per cent of people with TS have autism, though only a tiny percentage of people with autism have TS.

- *Gilles de la Tourette syndrome*: about 10 per cent of people with autism have vocal or motor tics, which are features of Tourette syndrome.

- *Smith-Lemli-Opitz Syndrome*: A genetic condition caused by a defect in cholesterol synthesis. About 75% of such children have autism.

- *Timothy Syndrome*: this rare condition caused by abonormalities in the calcium channel signalling system leads to a range of medical symptoms (e.g., cardiac arthythmia that can be fatal in childhood). 80% of children with Timothy Syndrome are said to also have autism. This has led to new interest in calcium channels in autism.

- *Duchenne Muscular Dystrophy*: This X-linked recessive degenerative neuromuscular disorder is caused by deficient dystrophin protein in the muscle. It is sometimes also associated with autism.

In summary, there is no longer any doubt that autism and Asperger syndrome are biological, and the challenge is in integrating the biology with the psychology of these conditions. Relating this evidence with ways of intervening is the subject of the final chapter of this book.

7

Intervention, education, and treatment

> **➔ Key points**
>
> Special education makes a difference, as does individual and family support. New treatments are heralded every year, and many of them turn out to be nothing more than hype. Be wary of following the latest fashion in treatment lest this turn out to be costly not only in terms of your family savings, but also in terms of your time and stress levels. The critical piece of advice is that when you read in the newspaper or on the web that there is a breakthrough new treatment or intervention for autism or Asperger syndrome, do not rush to take your child to get that treatment. Wait, look at http://www.researchautism.net, and be cautious.

There is a huge and potentially bewildering array of types of interventions either that are being used for people with autism and Asperger syndrome, or that are claimed to be useful. Parents and others need a single source of information where they can read unbiased accounts of these different interventions and can see the evidence for or against each one, so that they can make informed choices as to which intervention to follow.

Fortunately, the charity *Research Autism* has created a website (http://www. researchautism.net) which aims to list every known intervention, and gives each one a rating (from very good to very bad, and every shade in between). To get a very bad rating, the intervention has to be known to have unwanted side-effects or even be dangerous. Sadly there are a few such interventions. Some are simply being pushed hard for commercial reasons, and parents and others need to know if it is true that a specific intervention (let's call it X) really does help. This requires independent evidence obtained through systematic evaluation of intervention X compared with intervention Y, conducted in a scientifically rigorous manner. To get a good rating, the intervention would have been through such an evaluation and have been shown to have some benefits. To get a very good rating, this would be apparent across a number of independent studies.

What do we mean by a scientifically rigorous evaluation? Effectively we are talking about a 'treatment trial', which is common in the field of medical treatments but rare in the field of psychological, behavioural or educational interventions. Arguably it is just as important to know if drug X is beneficial or harmful as to know if psychological intervention X is beneficial or harmful (or just a waste of a family's savings).

The website mentioned above not only lists all the known interventions, but if you click on 'Advanced' you can read the list of studies that have evaluated each of these interventions. If you are so inclined, you can even follow the links to the scientific studies themselves, which are usually held in a medical database, such as *PubMed*. These list the journal articles that have been published on a particular topic, and which have been through 'peer review'. That should give parents and others more faith in the evaluation, because it is not just a commercial company saying 'Try treatment X' and it is not just a particularly passionate, charismatic clinician or scientist saying 'Try treatment X'. It is a report that has been through the sober checking process, checking that the evidence was collected in a way that conclusions can be drawn meaningfully and reasonably.

For non-scientists, it is worth listing the key features of a well-designed 'treatment trial'. These are things you can look for when evaluating the evidence for yourself:

* Were the people with autism or Asperger syndrome *randomly assigned* into two groups, one receiving X and one receiving Y?

* Were the two groups *matched* in important ways (age, IQ, social class, etc.) before being compared after a certain time-frame to see if people in group X were scoring better on some relevant measure, compared with those in group Y?

* Were there enough people in each group (this is the *sample size*) such that statistical tests could be properly used to compare the two groups? (A minimum sample size would be, as a rule of thumb, about 12 people in each group.)

(continued)

- Were the scientists who analysed the results (comparing the two groups) *blind* as to who was in which group?

- Were the participants *blind* as to the predictions of the researchers?

- In the case of a medical treatment, were the participants blind as to which treatment they were getting? If they were, and if the scientists were blind as to who was in which group, this is known as a *double-blind* treatment trial. In the case of a psychological or educational intervention, it may not be possible to keep the participants blind as to which kind of intervention they are receiving.

- Were the participants receiving any other interventions at the same time, such that we can conclude that any improvement in group X over group Y is really down to intervention X? This relates to whether there might be *confounding factors* that could equally well explain the effects.

Such treatment trials are hard to conduct and are expensive in terms of research funding. Typically, such a study would require a researcher with 3 years funding, to compare 20 children who had 'dolphin therapy' (as an example of one treatment which has been claimed to be helpful for autism) and 20 who simply went to a social skills group (in the same location e.g. California). This is to ensure the two groups were matched (e.g. in terms of coming from families who would take their child off to California for an intervention). As can be seen, such studies are complicated to complete. For this reason, not all interventions or treatments listed on the website above have yet been through a treatment trial. These features of a treatement trial are the ideal but may not always be attainable.

In this chapter, some of the more well-known interventions and treatments and educational methods are briefly described. Readers should consult the website at www.researchautism.net for an up-to-date and comprehensive list. The hope is that whereas this book will be a snapshot in time, that website will be continuously updated as new studies are published, so that it can be used as a resource for making informed decisions.

Non-specific interventions

Music therapy

There are many reports of the positive effects of music therapy. This may come as no surprise given that music is a system, and we saw in Chapter 5 how children with autism and Asperger syndrome like predictability and systematic or highly structured information. In addition, some children with autism or Asperger syndrome are actually very talented or intuitive when it comes to analysing, reproducing or producing music.

A famous example is the English young man Derek Paravacini, who not only has quite severe, classic autism but is also completely blind. Despite this double disability, he has stunned audiences around the world with his enormous repertoire of jazz songs that he plays on piano, obviously from memory. He improvised with boogie-woogie master Jools Holland at a concert in Cambridge in September 2006 (Figure 7.1), showing that he can use music to interact and react to novelty. He is clearly a *savant* in that his musical skills are way beyond his other skills. (He could not live independently, or indeed manage any part of his life, and needs total care and support to function.)

Whilst many people with autism or Asperger syndrome do not have a savant skill in this area, many of them may enjoy the repetition of music and find it

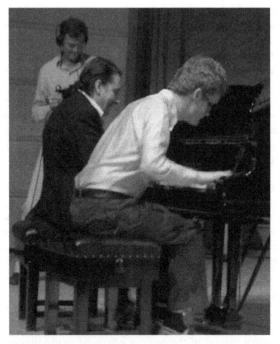

Figure 7.1 Derek Paravicini playing a duet with Jools Holland at the Cambridge Concert for Autism, West Road Concert Hall, September 2006.

an arena in which they can join in with others, even if only one-to-one. It can be a powerful way of teaching turn-taking, if the music session is designed with a dialogue-type structure. Whereas verbal conversational dialogue may be too difficult for some people with autism or Asperger syndrome, because of the open-endedness of small-talk and chatting, music may reduce the number of possible directions in which an interaction may go, because it is more rule governed. As a result, many schools for autism offer music therapy.

Art therapy

Art therapy is also now a widely available intervention in schools for children with autism or Asperger syndrome. Again, this is because it builds on an area of strength in autism spectrum conditions, since many people with autism spectrum conditions prefer to think visually than verbally. (Temple Grandin, a woman with autism who is an Associate Professor of Animal Science in Colorado State University, emphasizes such visual thinking in her book *Thinking in Pictures*.) Artistic skill can also be developed in a highly systematic way, such that some people with autism produce hundreds of the same kinds of drawings over and over again, until they have perfected a technique.

An example is from an Italian woman with autism, Lisa Perini, who as a child filled her notebook with repetitive productions such as that in Figure 7.2, but who as an adult now has total control over her pen and paintbrush, producing work such as that shown in Figure 7.3.

A different kind of example is from an English man with Asperger syndrome, Peter Myers, who uses a strongly systemizing approach to his art to produce highly detailed images which reveal both his understanding of illusion (Figure 7.4) and how carefully he can plan a whole piece of work (Figure 7.5).

Other autistic savants who are visual artists include Stephen Wiltshire (whose book *Cities* shows his strongly architectural and technical approach to art) and Gilles Tréhin whose book entitled *Urville* again shows his imagination in designing a virtual city along exquisitely detailed architectural and town-planning principles.

We should recognize that the majority of people with autism or Asperger syndrome have not developed their visual art skills to such a high level but may nevertheless enjoy art therapy as an opportunity to interact with another person without a strong verbal component, and to take pride in their work.

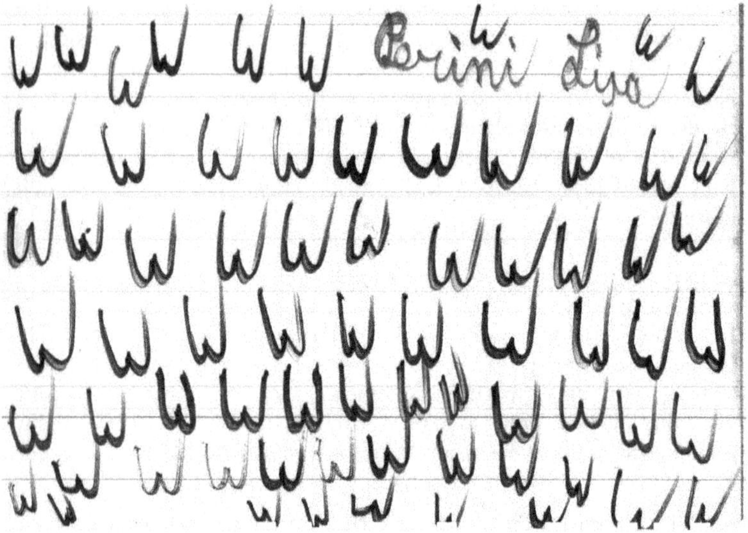

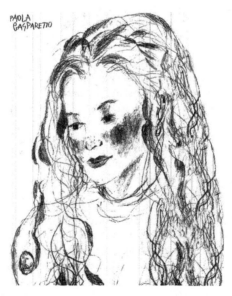

Figure 7.2 Repetitive patterns produced by Lisa Perini, as a child with autism.

Figure 7.3 Drawing by Italian artist Lisa Perini, now an adult with autism.

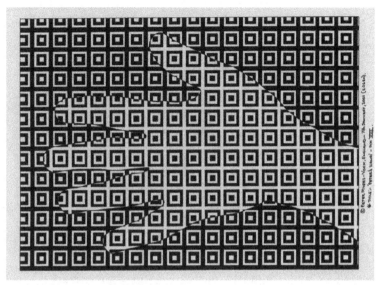

Figure 7.4 Peter's hand Mk VIII, by Peter Myers.

Speech and language therapy

Speech therapy is seen as a core part of the curriculum in schools for children with autism and Asperger syndrome. This is because in classic autism there is invariably language delay. Speech therapy may aim to minimize the size of the language delay. This is particularly important because the presence of language before age 5 years is a strong predictor of prognosis, as is language level in the toddler years.

Speech therapists typically do not focus just on words and verbal skills but also on social skills such as joint attention (pointing and gaze following). This is because joint attention is a building block for social skills (including mindreading or theory of mind) and communication. During joint attention, the child and adult establish a shared focus of attention on an object. In conversational terms this is equivalent to establishing a *topic*. There is little point in teaching words for things if the child has no idea about an object or event being a topic of communication. Speech therapists may also focus not just on a child's ability to increase their vocabulary (though this is important) but also on how language skills are used. This entails helping the child with *pragmatics*, or the social use of language.

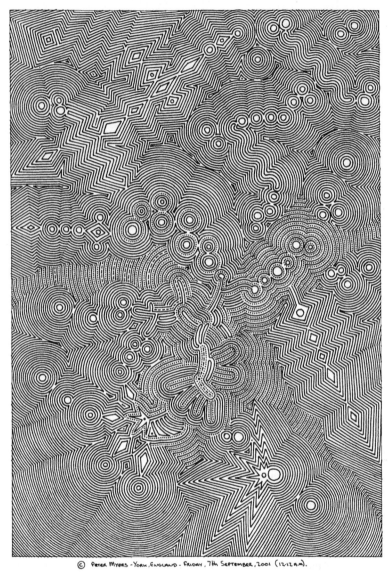

© Peter Myers - York, England - Friday, 7th September, 2001 (12·12 a.m.).

Figure 7.5 Circles, by Peter Myers.

Related to this will be helping the child understand non-literal language (such as metaphor, irony, humour, figurative language and sarcasm). These are the areas of language that depend on being able to understand not just the words actually spoken or written but also the *intentions* of the speaker (the intention to joke, for example), an area that even high-functioning children with autism or Asperger syndrome find difficult to grasp.

One young woman with Asperger syndrome, aged 27, who is doing a PhD, told me she had only just discovered that people do not always say what they mean. This came as a total shock to her and pushed her into a state of extreme anxiety, suddenly unable to rely on her grasp of word meanings. She had previously assumed that people's words were truthful and faithful references to objects or events. This is surprisingly late to discover this, as the typical 4-year-old who grasps deception and trickery already appreciates that what people say and what people mean may be two very different things.

Some speech therapists will teach *Makaton* (which uses a simplified core vocabulary of 450 concepts) or concentrate on using non-vocal systems of communication, such as sign language, if a child is making very little progress with spoken language. A well-evaluated method that is growing in use is the *Picture Exchange Communication System (PECS)*, whereby a picture is exchanged by a child, to request an object or activity that he or she wants. Its clear rules may be why it is very successful, since this taps into strong systemizing.

Educational services

Education remains the most important method of intervention for people on the autistic spectrum. This is true both for children who are very 'low functioning' and who may need to attend a special school or unit just for children with autism, or a child with Asperger syndrome who may need his or her own teaching support assistant to help him or her remain in a mainstream classroom, or may need to attend a special school or unit for children with Asperger syndrome. It is even true for adults with Asperger syndrome who are in further education and who need the college Disability Officer to assess and meet their own particular educational needs. Finally, adults with autism may need continuing education in daily life on social skills. Different schools have different educational philosophies.

Daily life therapy and occupational therapy

Daily Life Therapy approach puts an emphasis on group physical activities. The *Higashi School* in Boston is an example of a school that uses this. It remains unclear what the importance of this is, though taking the hyper-systemizing view of autism and Asperger syndrome it may be that structured group physical activities are an easier way to socialize than unstructured (free-play) social situations. A broader approach is occupational therapy, which has value in supporting the individual in a broader range of everyday activities.

Early intensive behavioural interventions

This approach focuses on shaping skills using rewards (based on what each individual child will 'work' to earn). One example of this is known as ABA (*Applied Behavioural Analysis*) and one version was evaluated by California-based psychologist Ivar Lovaas. *Treehouse* in London and the *Help Group* in Los Angeles are flagship examples of schools that advocate ABA.

The original ABA methods in the 1970s included punishment as well as reward (based on behavioural or learning theory). Fortunately the punishment element is no longer a feature of this teaching method. ABA is offered at home as well as in some schools, since some advocates of ABA believe that it needs to be 'around the clock', for as many as 40 hours per week per child. This requires a team of ABA therapists who can provide this continuity. It is not known if benefits might be apparent from fewer than 40 hours per week. Most studies find this approach beneficial.

TEACCH (Treatment and Education of Autistic and Communication-Handicapped Children)

This was developed in 1966 at the University of North Carolina by Eric Schopler. The name reflects its now rather outdated terminology, though the principles remain important. It emphasizes individual teaching programmes, social skills training, structured teaching, teaching generalization (an area of difficulty for many children with autism and Asperger syndrome) and *cognitive behaviour therapy* (in which principles from psychology are applied to autism). There is considerable evidence that structured approaches to teaching children with autism are helpful, especially when information is presented in an unambiguous and highly consistent format.

The Son-Rise programme ("Options")

This method was developed by Barry and Samahria Kauffman (parents of a child with autism called Raun) in the early 1980s, in New York. Following the success of their book and film, they set up the *Autism Treatment Center of America* which offers Son-Rise. It advocates a home-based one-to-one teacher-child relationship in which the teacher follows the child's lead. This is likely to be useful because many children with autism or Asperger syndrome can manage a one-to-one social relationship but have difficulties in unstructured social groups. Even in their one-to-one relationships, they prefer to be in control, so if the teacher is following the child's lead, this means the child will be less anxious. Further, rather than expecting the child with autism or Asperger syndrome to join the non-autistic world, the teacher makes the effort to join the autistic world. As such, it allows the child to be themselves, rather than insisting that they become different.

One criticism of this approach is that it might lead to the child remaining in a very autistic world. Against this one might imagine that building trust in one adult would enable the child with autism to learn a lot about the social world that they are avoiding. This could be seen as eventually leading the adult to be a trusted individual who can act as interpreter between the child's autistic world and the 'neurotypical' world, explaining it to the child much as an anthropologist entering a foreign culture relies on a trusted 'informant'. There are no formal evaluations of this method.

Social skills teaching and mindreading

At the core of most educational approaches to autism and Asperger syndrome is the teaching of social skills. Some do this via role-play and drama therapy, which can be challenging for some children with autism or Asperger syndrome. Some teach social skills in a more didactic fashion, teaching specific social *behaviours* (such as eye contact, not standing too close to another person, or not speaking so loudly) or specific social *rules* (such as holding the door open for other people, how long to hold on if the phone is ringing before someone answers, or how to reply if someone gives you a present). Such approaches can be very effective, but the risk is a rigid use of social skills since rules are hard to specify in a way that covers every instance. Some methods use the popular *Social Stories* method developed by Carol Gray which provides common social situations and teaches social scripts in order to help children learn what to expect in different situations.

A different approach focuses on teaching about *mental states* (beliefs, thoughts, intentions, desires and emotions) in order to help the individual develop a 'theory of mind' or *mindreading* skills. There are a variety of methods to do this. One method uses cartoon think-bubbles to make it explicit what others are thinking. Another method uses a manikin head and Polaroid photos to make it clear what another person can see. These methods are described in a book called *Teaching Children with Autism to Mind-read: A Practical Guide*, published in 1999 by Wiley. A controlled trial of this method suggests that children with autism can be taught to understand the basic principles relating mental states to behaviour (such as 'seeing leads to knowing', or 'people feel happy when the get what they want') and can even learn more complex principles, such as 'people feel happy if they *think* they are getting what they want').

Some educational software has attempted to teach the specific mindreading skill of emotion recognition. The DVD that does this is called *Mind Reading* (http://www.jkp.com/mindreading) which is an electronic encyclopedia of human expressions of emotions. It contains 412 different emotions, each portrayed on six different actors' faces and in their voices (male and female, old and young, different ethnicities). It includes examples suitable for very young children through to adulthood. This enables people with autism or Asperger syndrome to study emotions in a highly systematic way (harnessing their strong systemizing) much like someone might study a foreign language. Trials of both adults and children with Asperger syndrome show that using the DVD for as short a period as 10 weeks can lead to significant improvement in emotion recognition and, in the case of children, a degree of 'generalization' to material on which they were not trained (see Figure 7.6).

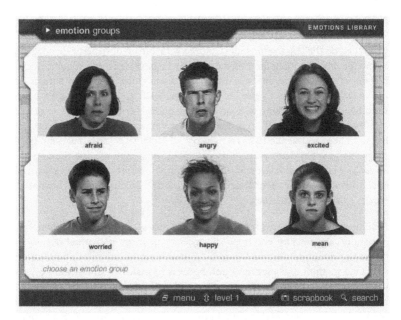

Figure 7.6 Examples of screen shots from *Mind Reading* (DVD).

An equivalent for pre-schoolers which has been developed is *The Transporters*. This is a children's animation series in which the main characters are vehicles that move in highly systematic ways (again, harnessing the strong interest in systems among even very young children with autism and Asperger syndrome) but where there are facial expressions of emotion 'grafted' onto the animated vehicles (www.transporters.tv) (see Figures 7.7 and 7.8).

Support agencies

Employment support

There is a growing recognition of the value of employment support agencies to help adults with high-functioning autism or Asperger syndrome find and keep a job. As an example, the National Autistic Society in the UK runs an agency called *Prospects* that helps adults with Asperger syndrome find employment. They first assess the strengths of the person with Asperger syndrome and help them prepare a curriculum vitae. They explain to a prospective employer that a conventional interview selection process may not bring out the best in the candidate but that in employing a person with Asperger syndrome they not only get a totally loyal, honest, straight-talking person, but they get someone who finishes tasks to a high level of detail, no matter how many hundreds of hours the task takes, and no matter how repetitive or routine the procedural aspects

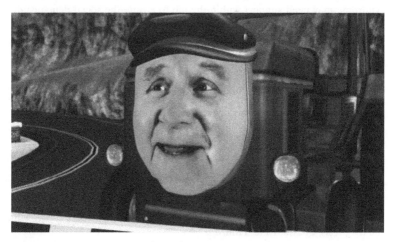

Figure 7.7 Barney's Happy Day: from *The Transporters*.

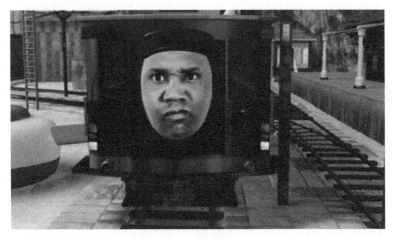

Figure 7.8 Charlie's Grumpy Day: from *The Transporters*.

of the task may be. Indeed, procedural repetition (a key part of systemizing) may even hold some attraction for a person with Asperger syndrome, whereas this might lead anyone else to 'cut corners'.

They also explain to an employer that the person with autism or Asperger syndrome may need support within the job to ensure the social demands do not become too great; that there may at times be crises if misunderstandings arise or if things are unpredictable; and that *Prospects* is there to come back in and help resolve such crises.

Befriending, advocacy, mentoring and social support groups

People with autism or Asperger syndrome may have difficulty making friends. Befriending schemes are a practical way to assist this. Students or employees with Asperger syndrome may also find it useful to have a mentor who can help them with practical planning in their everyday life. Social support groups may be a way for them to meet other people with a diagnosis so as not to feel isolated and to realize that they are not the only person struggling to find ways of coping. There are also support groups for parents, grandparents, siblings and partners, since autism spectrum conditions affect not just the individual with the diagnosis, but the wider family.

Medical treatments and diets

There are as yet no medical treatments for autism *per se*. It is important to note that the very idea of a medical treatment for autism or Asperger syndrome can in some cases be ethically controversial, since whilst some aspects of autism cause suffering and could benefit from alleviation, other aspects of autism simply represent a different way of processing information, need not interfere or cause suffering, and may even lead to talent.

If there were a medical treatment for the social and communication difficulties, this might well be desirable. If there were a medical treatment that helped the individual be more flexible, this too might be desirable. But a medical treatment that reduced the autistic tendency towards detailed perception or towards strong systemizing might be undesirable, as these are arguably areas of strength.

There have been trials using *antidepressants* including the SSRIs (selective serotonin reuptake inhibitors, such as fluoxetine [Prozac]), or the monoamine oxidase inhibitors (MAOIs) or tricyclics. These have shown some effect on certain features of behaviour, such as a reduction in repetitive behaviour. However, there are concerns about the use of these drugs in children because of the risk of inducing other side-effects (such as agitation). *Antipsychotic drugs* (also sometimes known as neuroleptics, including risperidone) have also been tried as a treatment for irritability and hyperactivity in autism or Asperger syndrome but again carry risks of side effects (such as weight gain, mood swings, drowsiness and raised serum prolactin levels).

Diets

Gluten free, casein free, yeast free

Casein is a protein found in milk and cheese. Gluten is a protein found in some cereals, particularly those with wheat, barley and rye. Some people suggest that these proteins are not properly digested in people with autism or Asperger syndrome and may cause allergies. Yeast-free diets are claimed to be useful for those children or adults with autism or Asperger syndrome who have gastrointestinal problems. There have been some trials of gluten- and/or casein- and/or yeast-free diets in autism, but these are inconclusive. Individual accounts by parents exist documenting improvements in the child's behaviour and, at times, deterioration. For this reason, any dietary intervention needs to be carefully monitored in case the withdrawal of a key element of a child's diet is leading to even greater difficulties.

Vitamin B6 supplements have been proposed as useful in autism, but the evidence is mixed. Vitamin B6 taken in higher dosage can lead to magnesium deficiency which is associated with bed-wetting (enuresis). Vitamin B15 (also known as DMG or dimethylglycine) has also been claimed to improve eye contact and speech, but it is also known that DMG can cause hyperactivity. As such, vitamin supplements such as these should only be considered under medical guidance, and their claims as treatments for autism or Asperger syndrome are not substantiated.

Horror stories

Over the years, there have been some treatments for autism that have been heralded as being a 'miracle cure'. Each has turned out not to be, and some have even caused suffering.

> *Secretin* is a gastrointestinal hormone involved in food digestion. In 1998, a boy with autism was given secretin and his parents reported an improvement in eye contact, smiling and sociability. This led to hundreds of families paying privately to have a course of treatment for their child. Whilst a few treatment trials showed some evidence of improvement, the majority did not, and the side effects can include high temperature, constipation and nausea.
>
> *Facilitated communication* involves a communicating partner who physically supports the individual to point to pictures, symbols, letters or words to communicate using a computer keyboard. It was claimed that individuals who had profound communication difficulties and no functional language could communicate fluently with facilitated communication. Systematic trials showed that it was the facilitator who produced the communication, not the individual. During the hype of the 1980s and 1990s, many families spent large amounts of money buying the special equipment. There were even allegations of physical abuse made through facilitated communication, as if these were first-hand testimonies, but which were being produced by the facilitator. Such allegations can rip a family apart.
>
> *Luprin/luprolide* is a drug to reduce testosterone, the so-called male hormone. A father and son team of clinicians (M. Geier and D. Geier) advocated the use of this anti-androgen for autism, even though it had
>
> (*continued*)

only been used to treat prostate cancer, precocious puberty, or to reduce sex drive in sexual offenders. The Geiers claimed that reducing testosterone in children with autism would help them excrete heavy metals such as mercury from the body that they claimed were building up in toxic levels. Following a detailed critique by parent Kathleen Seidel, the Geiers' published paper was retracted. Luprolide can have a number of serious side-effects, not just on sexual function, but causing testicular pain and painful urination. There is no good evidence that it is beneficial for autism.

Chelation is the other controversial medical procedure for reducing mercury levels that has been used in autism. It can cause liver and kidney damage, and, in the absence of convincing evidence that people with autism need mercury detoxification in the first place, this is not a treatment that should be pursued.

Parents of children with autism, and adults with high-functioning autism or Asperger syndrome, need to remain open-minded but sceptical about new 'treatments' that emerge, as they do each year. The best advice is to wait before rushing in to try the latest new method or treatment, until a range of studies are available, so that a balanced view of their costs and benefits can be reached.

It would be misleading to close on a note of concern. Although there is still a long way to go before we can say that people with autism or Asperger syndrome are well-supported in our society, we have come a long way in terms of both our understanding and our approaches. This book ends with a plea for even greater understanding, even more sensitive approaches, and a recognition that there is no room for complacency.

Endnotes

Chapter 1

1. The differences between classic autism and Asperger syndrome are shown visually in Figure 1.2. This plots both sub-groups on two dimensions (IQ and language onset). If you are at zero, this means you are average. More than 1 standard deviation (SD) above zero means above average, and more than 1 SD below zero means below average. As can be seen, classic autism occupies the space in the lower two quadrants, and Asperger Syndrome is located in the top right-hand quadrant. Some people suggest that people with Williams Syndrome (who have below average IQ but who are very chatty) might be the mirror image of classic autism, and would be located in the top left hand quadrant.

2. This is also sometimes referred to as Pervasive Developmental Disorder – Not Otherwise Specified (or PDD-NOS). The concept of 'autistic traits' is explained in Chapter 2.

Chapter 3

1. The 'Broader Autism Phenotype' (BAP) refers to people who have a significant number of autistic traits but not average enough to warrant a diagnosis. The score of 26 for first-degree relatives is estimated and is currently being confirmed by my colleague Sally Wheelwright.

Chapter 5

1. This does not mean that people with autism lack kindness or sympathy, and indeed autism is not the same as being a psychopath. These are quite different kinds of conditions.

2. This was an ingenious comparison, conducted because cameras take pictures of events even if the event is no longer current, whilst minds form beliefs about events even if the event is no longer current. Even if people with autism can solve the former (predicting the content of photos) they have difficulty solving the latter (predicting the content of someone's beliefs). This neatly shows the discrepancy between empathizing and systemizing.

Chapter 6

Research has studied children who had indeed been the victims of extreme neglect and deprivation: the Romanian orphans brought up in substandard institutions where children were tied to beds and given only the bare minimum for physical survival, but had little or no opportunity to develop attachments with affectionate carers. Such children had a disproportionate rate of classic autism. One simple-minded conclusion was that the neglect had caused autism. However, when such children were followed up after adoption into caring families, many of them showed a marked reduction in their autistic traits, i.e. they recovered to some extent. This may mean that what *resembled* autism in their extreme state of neglect was a form of *pseudo-autism.*, superficially similar but due to very different causes. A second complication is that some of these children may actually have had neurological conditions in the first place, including classic autism, which is why they had been abandoned into orphanages. So a simple model of cause and effect is not straight forward from these studies.

Further Reading

Attwood, T, (2006) *Asperger Syndrome*. Jessica Kingsley Ltd.

Baron-Cohen, S, (2003) *The Essential Difference: Men, Women, and the Extreme Male Brain*. Penguin/Basic Books.

Baron-Cohen, S, (1995) *Mindblindness: An Essay on Autism and Theory of Mind*. MIT Press.

Frith, U, (2003) *Autism: Explaining the Enigma*. Blackwell.

Frith, U, (1991) *Autism and Asperger Syndrome*. Cambridge University Press.

Gillberg, C, & Coleman, M, (2000) *The Biology of the Autistic Syndromes* Cambridge University Press.

Happe, F, (1996) *Autism: An introduction to psychological theory*. UCL Press.

Wing, L, (2003) *The Autistic Spectrum*. Robinson Publishing.

Appendix 1

The Autism Spectrum Quotient (AQ): Adult version

This is downloadable from http://www.autismresearchcentre.com

How to score the AQ: see p. 122.

How to fill out the questionnaire

Below are a list of statements. Please read each statement very carefully and rate how strongly you agree or disagree with it by circling your answer.

1.	I prefer to do things with others rather than on my own.	definitely agree	slightly agree	slightly disagree	definitely disagree
2.	I prefer to do things the same way over and over again.	definitely agree	slightly agree	slightly disagree	definitely disagree
3.	If I try to imagine something, I find it very easy to create a picture in my mind.	definitely agree	slightly agree	slightly disagree	definitely disagree
4.	I frequently get so strongly absorbed in one thing that I lose sight of other things.	definitely agree	slightly agree	slightly disagree	definitely disagree
5.	I often notice small sounds when others do not.	definitely agree	slightly agree	slightly disagree	definitely disagree
6.	I usually notice car number plates or similar strings of information.	definitely agree	slightly agree	slightly disagree	definitely disagree

7.	Other people frequently tell me that what I've said is impolite, even though I think it is polite	definitely agree	slightly agree	slightly disagree	definitely disagree
8.	When I'm reading a story, I can easily imagine what the characters might look like	definitely agree	slightly agree	slightly disagree	definitely disagree
9.	I am fascinated by dates.	definitely agree	slightly agree	slightly disagree	definitely disagree
10.	In a social group, I can easily keep track of several different people's conversations.	definitely agree	slightly agree	slightly disagree	definitely disagree
11.	I find social situations easy.	definitely agree	slightly agree	slightly disagree	definitely disagree
12.	I tend to notice details that others do not.	definitely agree	slightly agree	slightly disagree	definitely disagree
13.	I would rather go to a library than a party.	definitely agree	slightly agree	slightly disagree	definitely disagree
14.	I find making up stories easy.	definitely agree	slightly agree	slightly disagree	definitely disagree
15.	I find myself drawn more strongly to people than to things.	definitely agree	slightly agree	slightly disagree	definitely disagree
16.	I tend to have very strong interests which I get upset about if I can't pursue.	definitely agree	slightly agree	slightly disagree	definitely disagree
17.	I enjoy social chit-chat.	definitely agree	slightly agree	slightly disagree	definitely disagree
18.	When I talk, it isn't always easy for others to get a word in edgeways.	definitely agree	slightly agree	slightly disagree	definitely disagree
19.	I am fascinated by numbers.	definitely agree	slightly agree	slightly disagree	definitely disagree
20.	When I'm reading a story, I find it difficult to work out the characters' intentions.	definitely agree	slightly agree	slightly disagree	definitely disagree
21.	I don't particularly enjoy reading fiction.	definitely agree	slightly agree	slightly disagree	definitely disagree

22.	I find it hard to make new friends.	definitely agree	slightly agree	slightly disagree	definitely disagree
23.	I notice patterns in things all the time.	definitely agree	slightly agree	slightly disagree	definitely disagree
24.	I would rather go to the theatre than a museum.	definitely agree	slightly agree	slightly disagree	definitely disagree
25.	It does not upset me if my daily routine is disturbed.	definitely agree	slightly agree	slightly disagree	definitely disagree
26.	I frequently find that I don't know how to keep a conversation going.	definitely agree	slightly agree	slightly disagree	definitely disagree
27.	I find it easy to 'read between the lines' when someone is talking to me.	definitely agree	slightly agree	slightly disagree	definitely disagree
28.	I usually concentrate more on the whole picture, rather than the small details.	definitely agree	slightly agree	slightly disagree	definitely disagree
29.	I am not very good at remembering phone numbers.	definitely agree	slightly agree	slightly disagree	definitely disagree
30.	I don't usually notice small changes in a situation, or a person's appearance.	definitely agree	slightly agree	slightly disagree	definitely disagree
31.	I know how to tell if someone listening to me is getting bored.	definitely agree	slightly agree	slightly disagree	definitely disagree
32.	I find it easy to do more than one thing at once.	definitely agree	slightly agree	slightly disagree	definitely disagree
33.	When I talk on the phone, I'm not sure when it's my turn to speak.	definitely agree	slightly agree	slightly disagree	definitely disagree
34.	I enjoy doing things spontaneously.	definitely agree	slightly agree	slightly disagree	definitely disagree
35.	I am often the last to understand the point of a joke.	definitely agree	slightly agree	slightly disagree	definitely disagree
36.	I find it easy to work out what someone is thinking or feeling just by looking at their face.	slightly agree	definitely agree	slightly disagree	definitely disagree

37.	If there is an interruption, I can switch back to what I was doing very quickly.	definitely agree	slightly agree	slightly disagree	definitely disagree
38.	I am good at social chit-chat.	definitely agree	slightly agree	slightly disagree	definitely disagree
39.	People often tell me that I keep going on and on about the same thing.	definitely agree	slightly agree	slightly disagree	definitely disagree
40.	When I was young, I used to enjoy playing games involving pretending with other children.	definitely agree	slightly agree	slightly disagree	definitely disagree
41.	I like to collect information aboutcategories of things (e.g. types of car, types of bird, types of train, types of plant, etc.).	definitely agree	slightly agree	slightly disagree	definitely disagree
42.	I find it difficult to imagine what it would be like to be someone else.	definitely agree	slightly agree	slightly disagree	definitely disagree
43.	I like to plan any activities I participate in carefully.	definitely agree	slightly agree	slightly disagree	definitely disagree
44.	I enjoy social occasions.	definitely agree	slightly agree	slightly disagree	definitel disagree
45.	I find it difficult to work out people's intentions.	definitely agree	slightly agree	slightly disagree	definitely disagree
46.	New situations make me anxious.	definitely agree	slightly agree	slightly disagree	definitely disagree
47.	I enjoy meeting new people.	definitely agree	slightly agree	slightly disagree	definitely disagree
48.	I am a good diplomat.	definitely agree	slightly agree	slightly disagree	definitely disagree
49.	I am not very good at remembering people's dates of birth.	definitely agree	slightly agree	slightly disagree	definitely disagree
50.	I find it very easy to play games with children that involve pretending	definitely agree	slightly agree	slightly disagree	definitely disagree

How to score your AQ:

Score one point for each of the following items if you answered 'Definitely agree' or 'slightly agree':

1, 2, 4, 5, 6, 7, 9, 12, 13, 16, 18, 19, 20, 21, 22, 23, 26, 33, 35, 39, 41, 42, 43, 45, 46.

Score one point for each of the following items if you answered 'Definitely disagree' or 'slightly disagree':

3, 8, 10, 11, 14, 15, 17, 24, 25, 27, 28, 29, 30, 31, 32, 34, 36, 37, 38, 40, 44, 47, 48, 49, 50.

Simply add up all the points you have scored and obtain your total AQ score.

How to interpret your AQ score

- 0 - 10 = **low**.
- 11 - 22 = **average**. (Most women score about 15 and most men score about 17).
- 23 - 31 = **above average**.
- 32 - 50 = **very high**. (Most people with Asperger Syndrome or high functioning autism score about 35).
- 50 = **Maximum**.

Appendix 2

List of organizations supporting people with autism spectrum conditions and their families, across the world

Autism Europe
Rue Montoyer 39 bte 11
1000 Brussels, Belgium
Tel: +32 (0) 2 675 7505
Fax: +32 (0) 2 675 7270
Email: secretariat@autismeurope.org
Website: http://www.autismeurope.org

World Autism Organization
Calle Navaleno 9
28033, Madrid, Spain
Tel: +34 91 766 2222
Fax: +34 91767 0038
Email: international@APNA.es

AUSTRALIA

Australian Advisory Board on Autism Spectrum Disorders
c/o 41 Cook Street, Forestville
NSW 2087, Australia
Tel: +61 (0)2 8977 8300
Fax: +61 (0)2 8977 8399
Website: http://www.autismaus.com.au

New South Wales

Autism Spectrum Australia (Aspect)
41 Cook Street, Forestville,
NSW 2087, Australia
Tel: +61 (0)2 8977 8300
FREECALL: 1800 06 99 78
Fax: +61 (0)2 8977 8399
Email: contact@autismnsw.com.au
Website: http://www.autismnsw.com.au

Queensland

Autism Association Queensland
P.O. Box 354, Sunnybank Hills,
Queensland 4109, Australia
Tel: +61 (0)7 3273 0000
Fax: +61 (0)7 3273 8306
Email: admin@autismqld.co.au
Website: http://www.autismqld.com.au

South Australia

Autism SA
Street address: 3 Fisher Street
Myrtle Bank SA 5064
Postal address: PO Box 339 Fullarton SA 5063
Tel: +61 (0) 88 379 6976
Fax: +61 (0) 88 338 1216
Email: admin@autismsa.org.au
Website: http://www.autismsa.org.au

Tasmania

Autism Tasmania
PO Box 1552, Launceston
TAS 7250, Australia
Tel: +61 (0) 363 24 755
Email: autism@autismtas.org.uk
Website: http://www.autismtas.org.au

Victoria

Autism Victoria
Postal address: P.O. Box 235, Ashburton
Victoria 3147, Australia
Street address: 35 High Street, Glen Iris
Victoria 3146, Australia
Tel: +61 (0)3 9885 0533
Fax: +61 (0)3 9885 0508
Email: admin@autismvictoria.org.au
Website: http://www.autismvictoria.org.au

Autistic Citizens Residential & Resources Society of Victoria Inc
PO Box 3015, Ripponlea
Victoria, 3185, Australia
Tel: +61 (0)417 384 454
Email: dcoates@asd.org.au
Website: http://www.asd.org.au

Western Australia

Autism Association of Western Australia
Postal address: Locked Bag 9, Post Office
West Perth, WA 6872, Australia
Street address: 37 Hay Street
Subiaco 6008, Australia
Tel: +61 (08) 9489 98900
Fax: +61 (08) 9489 8999
Email: autismwa@autism.org.au
Website: http://www.autism.org.au

AUSTRIA

Österreichische Autistenhilfe
Eßelinggasse 13/3/11
A-1010 Wien, Austria.
Tel: +43 1 533 96 66
Fax: +43 1 533 78 47
Email: office@autistenhilfe.at
Website: http://www.autistenhilfe.at

BAHRAIN

Bahrain Society for Children with Behavioral and Communication Difficulties
Post Office Box 37304
Kingdom of Bahrain
Tel: +973 17 730960
Fax: +973 17 737227
For direct contact within the United States
Use the following Voice mail/Fax number: 1 (206) 350-3256
Email: autism@batelco.com.bh
Website: http://www.childbehavior.org

BANGLADESH

The Autism Welfare Foundation
House #428, Road #2
Baitul Aman Housing Society
Shyamoli, Dhaka
Tel: +880 812 1759 or +880 0189 447 233

BELGIUM

Association de Parents pour l'Epanouissement des Personnes Autistes (APEPA)
Rue LEANNE, 15 à 5000 Namur
Belgium
Tel: +32 (0)81 744 350
Fax: +32 (0)81 744 350
Email: apepa@skynet.be
Website: http://www.ulg.ac.be/apepa

Vlaamse Vereniging Autisme
Groot Begijnhof 14
B – 9040 Gent
Belgium
Tel: +32 (0)78 152 252
Fax: +32 (0)9 218 83 83
Email: wa@autismevlaanderen.be
Website: http://www.autismevlaanderen.be

BRAZIL

Associação de Amigos do Autista (AMA)
Rua do Lavapés, 1123
Cambuci 01519-000
São Paulo, SP
Brazil
Tel: + 55 (11) 3376 4400
Fax +55 (11) 23376 4403
Email: falecomaama@aqma.org.br
Website: http://www.ama.org.br

CANADA

Autism Society Canada
Box 22017, 1670 Heron Road
Ottawa, Ontario, K1V 0C2
Canada
Tel: +1 613 789 8943 or 1 866 476 8440 (toll free)
Fax: +1 613 789-6985
Email: info@autismsocietycanada.ca
Website: http://www.autismsocietycanada.ca

Main Provinces:

Alberta

Autism Society of Edmonton Area
#101, 11720 Kingsway Avenue, Edmonton, Alberta,
T5G 0X5, Canada
Tel: +1 780 453 3971
Fax: +1 780 447 4948
Email: autism@compusmart.ab.ca
Website: http://www.edmontonautismsociety.org

British Columbia

Autism Society of British Columbia
303-3701 East Hastings Street, Burnaby, British Columbia
V5C 2H6, Canada
Tel: +1 604 434 0880 or 1 888 437 0880 (toll free)
Fax: +1 604 434 0801
Email: info@autismbc.ca
Website: http://www.autismbc.ca

Manitoba

Autism Society Manitoba
825 Sherbrook Street, Winnipeg, Manitoba,
Canada, R3A 1M5
Tel: +1 204 783 9563
Fax: +1 204 783 9563
Email: asm@mts.net
Website: http://www.autismmanitoba.com

New Brunswick

Autism Society New Brunswick
30 Ealey Crescent, Riverview,
New Brunswick, E1B 1E6
Canada
Tel: +1 506 372 9011 or 1 888 354 9622 (toll free)
Fax: +1 506 372 9011
Email: autism@nbnet.nb.ca
Website: http://www.sjfn.nb.ca/community_hall/A/auti3200.html

Newfoundland

Autism Society of Newfoundland and Labrador
70 Clinch Court, St John's, Newfoundland
Postal address: PO Box 14078
St. John's, Newfoundland,
A1B 4G8, Canada
Tel: +1 709 722 2803
Fax: +1 709 722 4926
Email: info@autismsociety.nf.net
Website: http://www.autism.nf.net/

Northwest Territories

Autism Northwest Territories
4904 Matonabee Street, Yellowknife,
North West Territories, X18 1X8, Canada
Tel: +1 867 920 4206
Fax: +1 867 873 0235
Email: autism@hotmail.com

Nova Scotia

Autism Society of Nova Scotia
1456 Brenton Street,
Halifax Nova Scotia,
B3J 2K7, Canada
Tel: +1 902 429 5529
Email: society@autismcentre_ns.ca
Website: http://www.autismsocietynovascotia.ca/

Ontario

Autism Society Ontario
1179A King Street West,
Suite 004, Toronto, Ontario,
M6K 3C5, Canada
Tel: +1 416 246 9592
Fax: +1 416 246 9417
Email: available from website
Website: http://www.autismontario.com

Aspergers Society of Ontario
161 Eglinton Avenue East # 401
Toronto, Ontario M4P 1 JS
Canada
Tel: +1 416 651 4037
Fax: +1 416 651 1935
Email: info@aspergers.ca
Website: http://www.aspergers.ca

Quebec

Fédération québécoise de l'autisme
et des autres troubles envahissants du développement
65 rue de Castelnau Ouest, bureau 104
Montréal (Québec), Canada
H2R 2W3
Tel: +1 514 270 7386
Fax: +1 514 270 9261
Website: http://www.autisme.qc.ca

Yukon

Autism Yukon
508F Main Street, Whitehorse
Yukon, Y1A 2B9, Canada
Tel: +1 867 667 6406
Fax: +1 867 667 6408
Email: info@autismyukon.org
Website: http://www.autismyukon.org

CHILE

ONG Corporación Andalué
Serrano 317, San Francisco de Limache, Chile
Tel: +56 (33) 412160
Fax. +56 (33) 416674
Email: andalue@gmail.com

CHINA

Beijing Rehabilitation Association for Autistic Children (BRACC)
The No 6 Hospital attached to Beijing University
No 51 Huayuan Bei Road, Haidian District, Beijing,
100083, P.R.China
Tel: +86 10 6207 8248
Fax: +86 10 6202 7314
Email: barac@public.fhnet.cn.net
Website: http://www.autism.com.cn

CZECH REPUBLIC

Autistic
Kyselova 1189/24
182 00 Prague 8, Czech Republic
Tel: +42 0605 400 865
Email: autistic@volny.cz
Website: http://www.volny.cz/autistik

DENMARK

Landsforeningen Autisme
Kiplings Alle 42,
DK-2860 Søborg,
Denmark
Tel: +45 7025 3065
Fax: +45 7025 3070
Email: kontor@autismeforening.dk
Website: http://www.autismeforening.dk

EGYPT

The Egyptian Autistic Society
9 Road 215
Degla, Maadi
Cairo, Egypt
Tel: +20 (2) 519 9033
Fax: +20 (2) 519 7055
Website: http://www.autismegypt.com

FINLAND

Finish Association for Autism (FAAAS)
Junailijankuja 3
SF-00520, Helsinki
Finland
Tel: +358 9774 2770
Fax: +358 (0)9 772 7710
Email: etunimi.sukunimi@autismliitto.fi
Website: http://www.autismiliitto.fi/

FRANCE

Autisme France
Lot 110-111, Voiek – 460 Avenue de la Quiera
06370 Mouans Sartoux, France
Tel: +33 (0) 493 460 177
Fax: +33 (0) 493 460 114
Email: autisme.france@wanadoo.fr
Website: http://www.autismefrance.org

GERMANY

Bundesverband Hilfe für das autistische Kind,
Vereinigung zur Förderung autistischer Menschen e.V.
Bebelallee 141
22297 Hamburg
Germany
Phone: +49 (0)40 511 5604
Fax : +49 (0)40 511 0813
Email: info@autismus.de
Website: http://www.autismus.de

GREAT BRITIAN AND NORTHERN IRELAND

See United Kingdom

GREECE

Greek Society for the Protection of Autistic People
2 Athenas Street
105 51 Athens
Greece
Tel: +30 210 321 6550
Fax: +30 210 321 6549
Email: gspap@internet.gr

HONG KONG

Society for the Welfare of the Autistic Person (SWAP)
Room 210-214, Block 19
Shek Kip Mei Estate
Kowloon, Hong Kong
Tel: +852 2788 3326
Fax: +852 2788 1414
Email: info@swap.org.hk
Website: http://www.swap.org.hk

HUNGARY

Autisták Érdekvédelmi Egyesülete
Hungarian Autistic Society (HAS)
H-1066 Budapest
Jókai utca 2-4 II/8
Hungary
Tel: +36 1 301 9067/354 1073
Fax: +36 1 302 1094
Email: autist@interpont.hu or info@esoember.hu
Website: http://www.esoember.hu or http://www.autista.info.hu

ICELAND

Umsjónarfélag Einhverfra
Háaleitisbraut 13
108 Reykjavík
Iceland
Tel: +354 562 1590
Fax: +354 562 1526
Email: einhverf@vortex.is
Website: http://www.einhverfa.is

INDIA

Action for Autism
Sector 5 Jasola Institutional Area
Behind Sai Nikatan, New Delhi 110025
India
Tel: +91 11 6534 7422, 4054 0991, 4054 0992
Fax: +91 11 4054 0993
Email: autism@vsnl.com
Website: http://www.autism-india.org

INDONESIA

Autism Foundation of Indonesia
Jl. Buncit Raya no. 55
Jakarta Selatan 1270
Indonesia
Tel: +62 21 797 1945
Fax: +62 21 799 1355
Email: mbudhiman@yahoo.com

IRELAND

Irish Autism Action
41 Newlands, Mullingar,
Co. Westmeath.
Tel: +353 (0)44-9331609
Email: kevin1aa@ircom.net
Website: http://www.autismireland.ie

Irish Society for Autism
Unity Building, 16/17 Lower O'Connell St.
Dublin 1 Republic of Ireland
Tel: +353 (01) 874 4684
Fax: +353 (01) 874 4224
Email: autism@isa.iol.ie
Website: http://www.autism.ie

Asperger Syndrome Association of Ireland (ASPIRE)
Coleraine House, Carmichael House, Coleraine Street
Dublin 7, Ireland
Tel: +353 (0) 879 336 160
Fax: +353 (0) 1873 5283
Email: familysupport@aspire-irl.org
Website: http://www.aspire-irl.org

ISRAEL

The Israeli National Autism Association (ALUT)
Website: http://www.alut.org.il

ITALY

Autismo Italia
Via Spartaco, 30 20135 Milano
Italy
Tel: +39 (0)2 700 537 540
Fax: +39 (0)2 700 537 540
Email: info@autismoitalia.org
Website: http://www.autismoitalia.org

JAMAICA

Jamaica Autism Support Group
c/o YMCA, 21 Hope Street
Kingston 10, Jamaica, West Indies
Tel: +1 876 926 8081
Fax: +1 876 929 9387
Email: jasa.jm@gmail.com

JAPAN

Autism Society Japan
Da Vinci 2, 6F
Akashicho, Chuoku
Tokyo 104-0044 Japan
Tel: +81 33 545 3380
Fax : +81 33 545 3381
Email: asj@autism.or.jp
Website: http://www.autism.or.jp

KENYA

National Autistic Center – Kenya
At Acorn Special Tutorials
412 Gitanga Road Valley Arcade
P.O Box 21436 00505
Tel: +254 020 3864436 / 7
Cell: +44 0733 785234 0725 959137
Email: acorn@clubinternetk.com

KUWAIT

Kuwait Center for Autism
Al-Rodha, Block 2, Yousef Al-Abieh Street
PO Box 33425, Al-Rodha 73455
Kuwait
Tel: +965 254 0351
Fax: +965 254 0247
Email: kwautism@qualitynet.net
Website: http://www.q8autism.com or http://www.safat.com/aut.html

LEBANON

Lebanese Autistic Society
Mazrra Street facing Russian Embassy
PO Box 23476, Beirut, Lebanon
Tel: +961 1 817 900
Fax: +961 136 4433
Email: info@autismlebanon.org
Website: http://www.autismlebanon.org

LITHUANIA

Autist Care Society "Autista"
Fax:+370 45 500326
Email: autista@takas.lt
Website: http://www.geocities.com/autista_lt

LUXEMBOURG

Autisme Luxembourg
c/o Mme Da Silva-Coelho
33 Bvd Pierre Dupong
L-1410 Luxembourg
Tel: +352 408 266
Fax: +352 298 039
Email: administration@autisme.lu
Website: http://www.autisme.lu

MACEDONIA

Macedonian Scientific Society for Autism
Institute of Special Education and Rehabilitation
Faculty of Philosophy, University St. Cyril and Methodius
Bull. Krste Misirkov b.b., 1000 Skopje
Republic of Macedonia
Tel. +389 2 3116 520 (Ext.234)
Fax: +389 23118 143
E-mail: vladotra@fzf.ukim.edu.mk
Website: http://www.mnza.org.mk

MALAYSIA

National Autism Society of Malaysia (NASOM)
No. 4 Jalan Chan Chin Mooi, Off Jalan Pahang
53200, Malaysia
Tel: +60 3 4022 3744
Fax: +60 3 4022 4495
Email: nasom@streamyx.com
Website: http://www.nasom.org.my and http://www.nasom.my.diip.net

MOROCCO

Association des Parents et Amis d'Enfants Handicapes Mentaux
Avenue "9 Avril" No. 68
Maarif Casablanca
Marocco
Tel: +212 25 81 43/25 57 11

NAMIBIA

Autism Namibia
PO Box 5043
Windhoek, Namibia
Tel: +264 (0)92 461 224 561/2
Fax: +264 (0)92 6561 228 255
Email: petard@iway.na

THE NETHERLANDS

Nederlandse Vereniging voor Autisme
The Dutch Autism Society
Prof. Bronkhorstlaan 10
3723 MB Bilthoven
The Netherlands
Tel : +31 (0)30 22 99 800
Fax: +31 (0)30 26 62 300
Email: info@autisme-nva.nl
Website: http://www.autisme-nva.nl

Autism Association for Overseas Families in the Netherlands
Terbregselaan 42, 3055
RG, Rotterdam, The Netherlands
Email: mail@aaof.info
Wesbite: http://www.aaof.info

NEW ZEALAND

Autistic Association of New Zealand
1st Floor, 257 Lincoln Road
Addington, Christchurch
New Zealand
Postal address: PO Box 42052
Tower Junction, Christchurch 8149
New Zealand
Tel: 0800 AUTISM (288 476) / +64 3339 2627
Fax: +64 (0)3 3339 2649
Email: info@autismnz.org.nz
Website: http://www.autismnz.org.nz

Cloud 9 Children's Foundation (Asperger Syndrome)
PO Box 30979
Lower Hutt
New Zealand
Tel: +64 (0)4 920 9488
Email: foundation@entercloud9.com
Website: http://www.withyoueverystepoftheway.com

NORWAY

Autismeforeningen i Norge
Postboks 6726, Etterstad
0609 Oslo, Norway
Tel: +47 23 05 45 70
Fax: +47 23 05 45 61/51
Email: post@autismeforeingen.no
Website: ww2.autismeforeningen.no/

PAKISTAN

Website: http://www.autism.meetup.com/77

PHILIPPINES

Autism Society Philippines
Room 305 M&L Building
Kamias Road, Quezon City
Metro Manila, Philippines
Tel: +63 (2) 926 6941
Fax: +63 (2) 926 6941
Email: admin@autismsocietyph.org
Website: http://www.autismsocietyph.org

PORTUGAL

Portuguesa para as Perturba ções do Defenvolvimento e Autismo
Prolongamento Da Rua 1
Rua José Luis Garcia Rodrigues - Bairro Alto da Ajuda,
1300 LISBOA Portugal
Tel: +351 213 616 250
Fax: +351 21 361 6259
Email: info@appda-lisboa.org.pt
Website: http://www.appda-lisboa.org.pt/

ROMANIA

Autism Romania – Association of Parents of Children with Autism
Postal address: O.P. 22, C.P.225,
Bucharest, Romania.
Tel: +40 (0)21 311 5099
Fax: +40 (0)21 311 5099
Email: office@autismromani.ro or president@autismromania.ro
Website: http://www.autismromania.ro

SERBIA

Autism Society of Serbia
11000 Beograd, Gundulicev Venac 40
Serbia and Montenegro
Tel: +381 11 3391 051
Email: autismpr@eunet.yu
Website: http://www.autizam.org.yu

SINGAPORE

Autistic Association (Singapore)
Block 381, Clementi Avenue 5
01-398, Singapore 120381
Tel: +65 774 6649
Fax: +65 774 6957
Email: autism@singnet.sg
Website: web.singnet.com.sg/~autism

Autism Resource Centre (Singapore)
Pathlight School
No. 6 Ang Mo Kio Street 44
Singapore 569253
Tel: +65 6323 3258
Fax: +65 6323 1974
Email: arc@autism.org.sg
Website: http://www.autism.org.sg

SLOVAKIA

Spoločnos' na Pomoc Osobám s Autizmom (SPOSA)
National Autistic Society of Slovakia
PO Box 89, 81000, Bratislava
The Slovak Republic
Tel: +421 (0)915 703709
Email: sposa@changenet.sk
Website: http://www.sposa.sk

SOUTH AFRICA

Autism South Africa
Transvaal Memorial Institute, Gate 13
Cnr Joubert Street Ext & Empire Bramfontein, Republic of South Africa
Postal address: PO Box 84209
Greenside 2034, Republic of South Africa
Tel.: +27 (0)11 484 9909/9923
Fax: +27 (0)11 486 3171
Email: info@autismsouthafrica.org
Website: http://www.autismsouthafrica.org

SPAIN

Asociación de Padres de Niños Autistas (APNA)
Cl Navaleno 9
28033 Madrid
Spain
Tel: +34 91 766 22 22
Fax: +34 91 767 00 38
Email: apna@apna.es
Website: http://www.apna.es

Federación Asperger España
Calle Foncalad n°11, Escalera
Izquierda 8°B
Spain
Tel: +34 639 363 000
Fax: +34 956 163 980
Email: info@asperger.es
Website: http://www.asperger.es

SWEDEN

Riksföreningen Autism (RFA)
The National Autistic Society
Bellmansgatan 30
118 47 Stockholm
Sweden
Tel: +46 08 702 05 80
Fax: +46 08 644 02 88
Email: info@autism.se
Website: http://www.autism.se

Föreningen Asperger/HFA
The Asperger/HFA Society
Website: ashfa.cjb.net

SWITZERLAND

Autismus Schweiz
Rue de Lausanne 91
CH-1700 Fribourg
Switzerland
Tel. +41 (0)26 321 36 11
Fax +41 (0)26 321 36 15
Email: infodoc@autism.ch
Website: http://www.autismswiss.ch

TRINIDAD AND TABAGO (West Indies)

Autistic Society of Trinidad & Tobago
St Helena Village, Via Caroni Post Office
Trinidad, Republic of Trinidad & Tobago
West Indies
Tel: +1 868 669 0462
Fax: +1 768 669 0462
Office tel: +1 868 663 8397
Email: autism@gmail.com

UNITED KINGDOM

England

The National Autistic Society (NAS)
393 City Road
London
England EC1V 1NG
Tel: +44 (0) 20 7833 2299
Helpline: 0845 070 4004
Fax: +44 (0) 20 7833 9666
Email: nas@nas.org.uk
Website: http://www.autism.org.uk

Northern Ireland

Autism NI (PAPA)
Donard House, Knockbracken Healthcare Park
Saintfield Road, Belfast
Northern Ireland, BT8 8BH
Tel: +44 (0)28 90 401729
Helpline: 0845 055 9010
Fax: +44 (0)28 90 403467
Email: info@autismni.org
Website: http://www.autismni.org

Scotland

The National Autistic Society in Scotland
Central Chambers, 1st Floor
109 Hope Street, Scotland, G2 6LL
Tel: + 44 (0) 141 221 8090
Fax: + 44 (0) 141 221 8118
Email: scotland@nas.org.uk
Website: http://www.autism.org.uk/scotland.html

Scottish Society for Autism
Hilton House, Alloa Business Park
Whins Road, Alloa
Scotland, FK10 3SA
Tel: +44 (0)1259 720 044
Fax: +44 (0) 1259 720 051
Email: autism@autism-in-scotland.org.uk
Website: http://www.autism-in-scotland.org.uk

Wales

Autism Cymru
6 Great Darkgate Street
Aberystwyth, Ceredigion
Wales, SY23 1DE
Tel: +44 (0)1970 625 256
Fax: +44 (0)1970 639 454
Email: buv@autismcymru.org
Website: http://www.autismcymru.org

National Autistic Society Cymru
6-7 Village Way, Greenmeadow
Springs Business Park, Tongwynlais
Cardiff, CF15 7NE
Tel: +44 (0)2920 629 312
Fax: +44 (0)2920 629 317
Email: cymru@nas.org.uk
Website: http://www.autism.org.uk/cymru

UNITED STATES OF AMERICA

Autism Society of America
7910 Woodmont Avenue
Suite 300, Bethesda
Maryland 20814, USA
Tel: +1 301 657 0881
Tel: 1 800 3AUTISM
Fax: +1 301 657 0869
Email: info@autism-society.org or chapters@autism-society.org
(for local chapters)
Website: http://www.autism-society.org

VENEZUELA

Venezuelan Society for Children and Adults with Autism
Avenida Alfredo Jahn con 3ra Trans
Quinta EMAUS.
Urbanización Los Chorros
Caracas 1071, Venezuela
Phone: +58 0212 237 1051/234 2536
Fax: +58 0212 2387339
Email: lnegron@sovenia.com.ve
Website: http://www.sovenia.com.ve

March 2008
Date information confirmed

Index